Heart Disease Prevention

Treatment, Recovery, and Lifestyle

Phillip J. Richmond

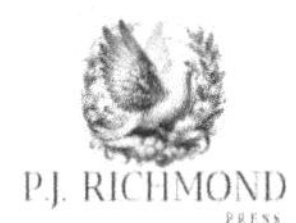

P.J. RICHMOND
PRESS

Dedication

To all the brave hearts battling heart disease, your resilience is the pulse that inspires this book. To the caregivers, your unwavering support is the rhythm that gives it life. And to the medical professionals, your dedication fuels the hope that beats within these pages. This book is a testament to your collective strength and courage.

Also By Phillip J. Richmond

Overcoming Trauma From Rape

How to Stop Masturbation

Breaking Free

The Problem of Grief

How to Be A Better Partner

Quick Wit, Confident Speech

Arthritis Pain Relief

Contents

Dedication...**3**

Introduction..**7**

Chapter 1: Treatment.....................................**13**

Types and Diagnosis of Heart Disease.............................14

Medical and Surgical Treatments for Heart Disease............17

Pros and Cons of Each Treatment Option.........................21

Potential Complications and Side Effects of Treatment........24

Best Practices and Tips for Following Your Treatment Plan....27

Chapter 2: Recovery.......................................**33**

The physical and emotional challenges of recovering

from heart disease...33

The importance of cardiac rehabilitation and follow-up care...........36

The lifestyle changes and adjustments you need to make after

treatment..41

The coping strategies and support resources for recovery..............57

The success stories and testimonials of heart disease

survivors...64

Chapter 3: Lifestyle.......................................**75**

The Role of Diet and Nutrition.......................................75

The Recommended Foods and Supplements.......................78

The Practical and Delicious Recipes and Meal Plans........................ 83

The Role of Exercise and Physical Activity..................................... 89

The Suitable and Enjoyable Exercises and Activities........................ 91

Chapter 4: Prevention.. 97

The Key Habits and Behaviors that Can Prevent or

Reduce the Risk of Heart Disease... 98

The Effective and Proven Ways to Quit Smoking, Lower Blood

Pressure, and Control Cholesterol... 111

The Stress Management and Relaxation Techniques

that Can Protect Your Heart... 129

The Importance of Regular Check-ups and Screenings for Heart

Disease... 136

The Future Trends and Innovations in Heart

Disease Prevention.. 142

Special Bonus.. 161

Introduction

Hello, and welcome to Heart Disease Prevention: Treatment, Recovery, and Lifestyle. My name is Phillip J. Richmond, and I am a health journalist and author. In this book, I will share with you the insights and advice I gained from interviewing one of the leading experts in the field of cardiology, Dr. Simon R. Kushi.

Dr. Kushi is a board-certified cardiologist and the director of the Heart Center at the Fortis Memorial Research Institute, Gurgaon. He has over 20 years of experience in treating patients with various forms of heart disease, from coronary artery disease to heart failure. He is also a passionate advocate for preventive cardiology, which is the branch of medicine that focuses on preventing heart disease before it develops or worsens.

I met Dr. Kushi when I was assigned to write a feature story about him and his work for a health magazine. I was intrigued by his approach to cardiology, which combines the best of conventional and alternative medicine. He believes that heart disease is not only a physical problem, but also a psychological, emotional, and spiritual one. He treats his patients holistically, addressing not only their symptoms but also their root causes and underlying issues.

As a journalist, I was curious to learn more about his methods and results. As a person, I was concerned about my own heart health, as I had a family history of heart disease. My father died of a heart attack when he was 52, and my mother suffered from angina and hypertension. I wanted to know how I could prevent heart disease, or at least delay its onset and complications.

I asked Dr. Kushi if he would be willing to share his knowledge and experience with me, and he graciously agreed. He invited me to visit his clinic and observe his practice. He also agreed to answer my questions and explain the concepts and principles of preventive cardiology. He was generous with his time and patient with my inquiries. He was also candid and honest about the challenges and limitations of his field.

Over the course of several weeks, I learned a lot from Dr. Kushi. I learned about what heart disease is and why it is important to prevent it. I learned about the main risk factors and causes of heart disease, and how to assess and reduce them. I learned about the common signs and symptoms of heart disease, and how to recognize and respond to them. I learned about the benefits of preventing and treating heart disease, both for my health and my quality of life. I also learned about the role of lifestyle in preventing and treating heart disease, and how to make positive changes to improve my heart health.

I was impressed by Dr. Kushi's expertise and wisdom, as well as his compassion and humility. He inspired me to take charge of my heart health, and to help others do the same. He also encouraged me to write this book, and to share his insights and advice with a wider audience. He said that he hoped that this book would help people understand and appreciate the importance of preventive cardiology, and to apply its principles and practices in their own lives.

Heart disease is a term that encompasses a range of conditions that affect the heart and blood vessels, such as coronary artery disease, heart attack, stroke, heart failure, arrhythmia, and congenital heart defects. According to the

World Health Organization, heart disease is the leading cause of death globally, accounting for nearly 18 million deaths in 2016. Moreover, heart disease is a major contributor to disability, reduced quality of life, and increased healthcare costs.

The good news is that heart disease can be prevented, treated, and even reversed in many cases. By adopting a healthy lifestyle, such as eating a balanced diet, exercising regularly, quitting smoking, managing stress, and controlling blood pressure and cholesterol levels, you can significantly lower your risk of developing heart disease or having a cardiac event. Furthermore, if you have been diagnosed with heart disease or have suffered a heart attack or stroke, you can still improve your condition and prevent further complications by following your doctor's advice, taking your medications, and making positive changes in your habits.

In this book, you will learn everything you need to know about heart disease prevention, treatment, recovery, and lifestyle. You will discover:

- The main risk factors and causes of heart disease, such as genetics, age, gender, ethnicity, smoking, obesity, diabetes, hypertension, high cholesterol, physical inactivity, and stress.

- The common signs and symptoms of heart disease, such as chest pain, shortness of breath, palpitations, dizziness, fatigue, nausea, and sweating.

- The different types and classifications of heart disease, such as ischemic, valvular, inflammatory, and congenital heart disease, and how they affect the structure and function of the heart and blood vessels.

- The various diagnostic tests and procedures that are used to detect and evaluate heart disease, such as electrocardiogram, echocardiogram, angiogram, stress test, and cardiac catheterization.

- The current treatment options and guidelines for managing heart disease, such as medications, surgery, stents, pacemakers, defibrillators, and cardiac rehabilitation.

- The best practices and recommendations for preventing and reducing the recurrence of heart disease, such as dietary modifications, physical activity, weight management, smoking cessation, blood pressure and cholesterol control, and stress management.

- The latest research and innovations in the field of heart disease, such as stem cell therapy, gene therapy, artificial organs, and nanotechnology.
- The practical tips and advice for living well with heart disease, such as coping with emotions, communicating with your healthcare team, finding support, and planning for the future.

By reading this book, you will gain a comprehensive and in-depth understanding of heart disease and how to prevent and treat it effectively. You will also learn how to enhance your well-being and enjoy a fulfilling and productive life despite having heart disease. Whether you are at risk of developing heart disease, have been diagnosed with it, or have survived a cardiac event, this book will provide you with valuable information, guidance, and inspiration to help you achieve optimal heart health and happiness.

Chapter 1: Treatment

If you have been diagnosed with heart disease, you may feel overwhelmed, scared, or confused. You may wonder what your diagnosis means, how it will affect your life, and what you can do to improve your condition. You may also have many questions about the different types of treatment options available, their benefits and risks, and how to choose the best one for you.

The goal of this chapter is to provide you with clear and comprehensive information about the treatment of heart disease. You will learn about the different types of heart disease and how they are diagnosed, the available medical and surgical treatments for heart disease, the pros and cons of each treatment option, the potential complications and side effects of treatment, and the best practices and tips for following your treatment plan. By reading this chapter, you will gain a better understanding of your condition and the various ways to treat it effectively. You will also feel more confident and empowered to make informed decisions about your health and well-being.

Types and Diagnosis of Heart Disease

Heart disease is a broad term that covers a range of conditions that affect the heart and blood vessels. The most common types of heart disease are:

1. Ischemic heart disease: This occurs when the arteries that supply blood to the heart muscle become narrowed or blocked by plaque, a fatty substance that builds up on the inner walls of the arteries. This reduces the blood flow and oxygen to the heart, causing chest pain (angina), shortness of breath, and irregular heartbeat (arrhythmia). If the plaque ruptures, it can form a blood clot that completely blocks the artery, leading to a heart attack (myocardial infarction) or sudden cardiac death.

2. Valvular heart disease: This occurs when one or more of the four valves that regulate the blood flow through the heart become damaged or defective. This can cause the valves to leak (regurgitate), narrow (stenose), or not close properly (prolapse). This affects the efficiency and function of the heart, causing symptoms such as fatigue, swelling, palpitations, and fainting. If left untreated, valvular heart disease can lead to heart failure, stroke, or infection (endocarditis).

3. Inflammatory heart disease: This occurs when the heart muscle (myocardium) or the membrane that surrounds the heart (pericardium) becomes inflamed due to an infection, autoimmune disorder, or other cause. This can cause chest pain, fever, and fluid accumulation around the heart (pericardial effusion). If the inflammation is severe, it can damage the heart muscle, causing heart failure, arrhythmia, or shock.

4. Congenital heart disease: This occurs when the heart or blood vessels are not formed correctly before birth, resulting in structural defects or abnormalities. These can affect the size, shape, or function of the heart or blood vessels, causing problems such as abnormal blood flow, low oxygen levels, or heart failure. Some examples of congenital heart defects are atrial septal defect (ASD), ventricular septal defect (VSD), patent ductus arteriosus (PDA), coarctation of the aorta, and tetralogy of Fallot.

The diagnosis of heart disease is based on your medical history, physical examination, and various tests and procedures that can assess the structure and function of your heart and blood vessels. Some of the common tests and procedures are:

1. Electrocardiogram (ECG or EKG): This is a simple and painless test that records the electrical activity of your heart. It can detect abnormal rhythms, signs of ischemia, damage, or enlargement of the heart, and the effects of medications or devices on the heart.

2. Echocardiogram: This is a test that uses sound waves (ultrasound) to create a moving picture of your heart. It can show the size, shape, and movement of your heart and its valves, chambers, and walls. It can also measure the blood flow and pressure in your heart and blood vessels, and detect any defects or abnormalities.

3. Angiogram: This is a test that uses a special dye and X-rays to show the inside of your arteries. It can reveal any blockages,narrowings, or abnormalities in your coronary arteries or other blood vessels. It can also measure the blood pressure and flow in your arteries.

4. Stress test: This is a test that measures how your heart works under physical stress, such as exercise or medication. It can show how well your heart pumps blood, how much oxygen your heart needs, and how your heart responds to increased demand. It can also detect any signs of ischemia, arrhythmia, or heart failure.

5. Cardiac catheterization: This is a procedure that involves inserting a thin, flexible tube (catheter) into a blood vessel, usually in your groin, arm, or neck, and guiding it to your heart or coronary arteries. It can perform various functions, such as measuring the pressure and oxygen levels in your heart chambers and blood vessels, taking samples of blood or heart tissue, injecting dye to perform an angiogram, or delivering treatments such as angioplasty or stenting.

Medical and Surgical Treatments for Heart Disease

The treatment of heart disease depends on the type, severity, and cause of your condition, as well as your overall health, age, and preferences. The main goals of treatment are to relieve your symptoms, improve your heart function, prevent or reduce the risk of complications, and enhance your quality of life. The treatment options can be divided into two categories: medical and surgical.

Medical Treatments

Medical treatments are those that involve the use of medications, devices, or lifestyle changes to treat your heart disease. Some of the common medical treatments are:

1. **Medications**: There are various types of medications that can help treat different aspects of heart disease, such as lowering blood pressure, cholesterol, or blood sugar levels, preventing blood clots, reducing inflammation, relieving pain, improving blood flow, regulating heart rate or rhythm, or strengthening the heart muscle. Some examples of medications are beta blockers, calcium channel blockers, angiotensin-converting enzyme (ACE) inhibitors, angiotensin II receptor blockers (ARBs), statins, aspirin, antiplatelets, anticoagulants, nitrates, diuretics, anti-inflammatories, anti-arrhythmics, and inotropes.

2. **Devices**: There are various types of devices that can help monitor, support, or correct your heart function, such as

pacemakers, implantable cardioverter defibrillators (ICDs), cardiac resynchronization therapy (CRT) devices, ventricular assist devices (VADs), or artificial hearts. These devices can be implanted or worn externally, and can deliver electrical impulses, mechanical assistance, or blood circulation to your heart or blood vessels.

3. Lifestyle changes: There are various types of lifestyle changes that can help prevent, manage, or improve your heart disease, such as quitting smoking, eating a healthy diet, exercising regularly, managing stress, limiting alcohol intake, maintaining a healthy weight, and following your treatment plan. These changes can help lower your risk factors, improve your symptoms, and enhance your well-being.

Surgical Treatments

Surgical treatments are those that involve the use of surgery or minimally invasive procedures to treat your heart disease. Some of the common surgical treatments are:

1. Angioplasty: This is a procedure that involves inserting a catheter with a balloon at its tip into a blocked or narrowed artery, and inflating the balloon to compress the plaque and widen the artery. This improves the blood flow and oxygen to the heart, and relieves chest pain or angina. A small metal mesh tube (stent) may be inserted into the artery to keep it open and prevent it from narrowing again.

2. Coronary artery bypass grafting (CABG): This is a surgery that involves taking a healthy blood vessel from another part of your body, such as your leg, arm, or chest, and attaching it to your heart to create a new route for blood to flow around a blocked or narrowed artery. This restores the blood supply and oxygen to the heart, and relieves chest pain or angina. This surgery can be done through a large incision in your chest (open-heart surgery) or through smaller incisions using special instruments (minimally invasive surgery).

3. Valve repair or replacement: This is a surgery that involves repairing or replacing a damaged or defective heart valve with a new one. The new valve can be made of biological tissue (from a human, animal, or synthetic source) or mechanical material (metal or plastic). This surgery can be done through a large incision in your chest (open-heart surgery) or through smaller incisions using special instruments (minimally invasive surgery) or a catheter (transcatheter surgery).

4. Heart transplant: This is a surgery that involves removing your diseased heart and replacing it with a healthy one from a donor. This surgery is done when your heart is severely damaged or failing, and other treatments have not worked or are not suitable for you. This surgery requires lifelong medication to prevent your body from rejecting the new heart, and regular follow-up care to monitor your heart function and health.

Pros and Cons of Each Treatment Option

Each treatment option for heart disease has its own pros and cons, and the best option for you may depend on various factors, such as your type and severity of heart disease, your overall health, your age, your preferences, and your doctor's recommendations. Here are some of the general pros and cons of each treatment option:

Medical Treatments

Pros:

- They are usually less invasive, risky, and costly than surgical treatments.
- They can help control your symptoms, improve your heart function, and prevent or reduce the risk of complications.
- They can be adjusted or changed according to your condition and response.
- They can be combined with other treatments, such as lifestyle changes or surgery, to enhance their effectiveness.

Cons:

- They may not work for everyone or for every type of heart disease.
- They may have side effects or interactions with other medications or supplements you are taking.
- They may require regular monitoring, testing, or follow-up visits to check your progress and adjust your dosage or regimen.

- They may require you to follow certain rules or restrictions, such as avoiding certain foods, drinks, or activities, or taking your medications at specific times or intervals.

Surgical Treatments

Pros:

- They can provide a more permanent or definitive solution for some types of heart disease, such as blocked arteries, damaged valves, or severe heart failure.
- They can restore or improve your heart function, blood flow, and oxygen levels, and relieve your symptoms more effectively than medical treatments in some cases.
- They can prevent or reduce the risk of serious or life-threatening complications, such as heart attack, stroke, or sudden cardiac death.

Cons:

- They are usually more invasive, risky, and costly than medical treatments.

- They may require general anesthesia, hospitalization, and a longer recovery time.
- They may have complications or side effects, such as bleeding, infection, scarring, or rejection of the new heart or valve.
- They may not work for everyone or for every type of heart disease.
- They may not eliminate the need for medications or lifestyle changes, and may require additional treatments or procedures in the future.

Potential Complications and Side Effects of Treatment

Although the treatment of heart disease can improve your condition and prevent or reduce the risk of complications, it may also have some potential complications and side effects that you should be aware of. These may vary depending on the type, severity, and cause of your heart disease, the type and duration of your treatment, your overall health, and your individual response. Some of the possible complications and side effects are:

1. Bleeding: This may occur during or after a surgery or procedure, such as angioplasty, CABG, valve repair or replacement, or heart transplant. It may also occur as a result of taking medications that thin your blood, such as antiplatelets or anticoagulants. Bleeding may be mild or severe, and may require transfusion, surgery, or medication to stop it. Bleeding may cause symptoms such as bruising, swelling, pain, or weakness.

2. Infection: This may occur due to exposure to bacteria, viruses, fungi, or other microorganisms during or after a surgery or procedure, such as CABG, valve repair or replacement, or heart transplant. It may also occur as a result of having a weakened immune system due to your heart disease or medications. Infection may affect your heart, blood vessels, or other organs, and may cause symptoms such as fever, chills, redness, swelling, pus, or drainage. Infection may require antibiotics, surgery, or other treatments to clear it.

3. Arrhythmia: This may occur due to damage or irritation to your heart muscle or electrical system during or after a surgery or procedure, such as angioplasty, CABG, valve repair or replacement, or heart transplant. It may also occur as a result of having an underlying heart condition, such as ischemic heart disease, valvular heart disease, or congenital heart disease. Arrhythmia may cause your heart to beat too fast, too slow, or irregularly, and may cause symptoms such as palpitations, dizziness, fainting, or chest pain. Arrhythmia may require medications, devices, or procedures to correct it.

4. Rejection: This may occur if your body's immune system attacks the new heart or valve that you received from a donor during a heart transplant or valve replacement. Rejection may occur soon after the surgery or procedure, or months or years later. Rejection may cause your new heart or valve to fail, and may cause symptoms such as fatigue, shortness of breath, swelling, fever, or weight gain. Rejection may require medications, devices, or procedures to treat it.

5. Side effects: These may occur as a result of taking medications or using devices to treat your heart disease. Side effects may vary depending on the type, dose, and duration of your treatment, your overall health, and your individual response. Side effects may be mild or severe, and may include nausea, vomiting, diarrhea, constipation, headache, drowsiness, dizziness, rash, itching, cough, or difficulty breathing. Side effects may require adjustment, change, or discontinuation of your treatment, or additional medications or treatments to manage them.

If you experience any of these complications or side effects, or any other unusual or bothersome symptoms, you should contact your doctor or health care team as soon as possible. They can help you identify the cause, assess the severity, and provide the appropriate treatment or intervention. They can also advise you on how to prevent or reduce the risk of these complications or side effects in the future.

Best Practices and Tips for Following Your Treatment Plan

Following your treatment plan is essential for the success of your treatment and the improvement of your heart disease. Your treatment plan is designed to suit your specific condition, needs, and goals, and to provide you with the best possible outcomes. Your treatment plan may include medications, devices, surgery, procedures, lifestyle changes, or a combination of these. To follow your treatment plan effectively, you should:

1. Understand your treatment plan: You should have a clear and comprehensive understanding of your treatment plan, including the purpose, benefits, risks, and expected results of each component of your treatment. You should also know how to use, take, or apply your medications or devices correctly, how to prepare for or recover from your surgery or procedure, and how to make or maintain your lifestyle changes. You should ask your doctor or health care team any questions or concerns you have about your treatment plan, and seek clarification or explanation if you are unsure or confused about anything.

2. Follow your treatment plan: You should follow your treatment plan as prescribed or instructed by your doctor or health care team. You should not skip, miss, or change your medications or devices without consulting your doctor or healthcare team. You should not delay or cancel your surgery or procedure without a valid reason or approval from your doctor or health care team. You should not ignore or disregard your lifestyle changes or recommendations without good justification or permission from your doctor or health care team. You should adhere to your treatment plan as closely and consistently as possible, and report any difficulties or challenges you face in following your treatment plan to your doctor or healthcare team.

3. Monitor your treatment plan: You should monitor your treatment plan regularly and carefully, and keep track of your progress and results. You should use tools or methods, such as a diary, a calendar, a checklist, or an app, to record or remind you of your medications, devices, surgery, procedures, or lifestyle changes. You should also measure or check your vital signs, such as your blood pressure, heart rate, weight, or blood sugar levels, as advised by your doctor or health care team. You should also note or document any symptoms, changes, or improvements you experience or observe in your condition, well-being, or quality of life. You should share or discuss your monitoring results with your doctor or health care team at your regular follow-up visits or appointments, or whenever necessary or requested.

4. Evaluate your treatment plan: You should evaluate your treatment plan periodically and objectively, and assess its effectiveness and suitability for your condition, needs, and goals. You should compare your current situation, status, and outcomes with your previous or expected ones, and identify any gaps, discrepancies, or problems. You should also consider any feedback, suggestions, or recommendations from your doctor or healthcare team, as well as any new or updated information or evidence about your treatment options. You should then decide if your treatment plan is working well for you, or if it needs any adjustment, modification, or change. You should communicate or consult with your doctor or health care team about your evaluation results, and collaborate with them to make any necessary or desired changes to your treatment plan.

By following these best practices and tips, you can follow your treatment plan effectively and efficiently, and achieve optimal results and benefits from your treatment. You can also prevent or reduce the risk of complications or side effects, and enhance your satisfaction and compliance with your treatment. You can also improve your condition and well-being, and enjoy a better and longer life with heart disease.

Choosing healthy foods and drinks is crucial. A diet rich in fruits, vegetables, whole grains, and lean proteins can help maintain a healthy weight and lower cholesterol and blood pressure levels

Chapter 2: Recovery

Recovering from heart disease is not easy. It can be a long and difficult process that affects not only your physical health, but also your emotional well-being, your relationships, your work, and your lifestyle. let's explore the various aspects of recovery, and how you can overcome the challenges and achieve a better quality of life after a heart attack, heart failure, or other heart problems.

The physical and emotional challenges of recovering from heart disease

Heart disease can cause serious damage to your heart muscle, blood vessels, and valves. Depending on the type and severity of your condition, you may need surgery, medication, or other treatments to restore or improve your heart function. These treatments can save your life, but they can also have side effects and complications that can affect your recovery.

Some of the physical challenges you may face after a heart attack or heart surgery include:

- Chest pain, discomfort, or tightness.
- Shortness of breath, fatigue, or weakness.
- Swelling in your legs, ankles, or feet.
- Irregular heartbeat, palpitations, or arrhythmia.
- Infection, bleeding, or wound-healing problems.
- Nausea, vomiting, or loss of appetite.
- Constipation, diarrhea, or other digestive issues.
- Sexual dysfunction or reduced libido.

These symptoms may be temporary or chronic, depending on your condition and treatment. They may also vary in intensity and frequency, depending on your activity level, stress, and other factors. You should always consult your doctor if you experience any of these symptoms, especially if they are new, severe, or persistent. Your doctor may adjust your medication, recommend additional tests, or refer you to a specialist if needed.

In addition to the physical challenges, you may also face emotional challenges after a heart attack or heart surgery. These include:

- Anxiety, fear, or worry about your health, your future, or your loved ones.
- Depression, sadness, or hopelessness about your situation or your recovery.
- Anger, frustration, or resentment about your condition or your treatment.
- Guilt, shame, or regret about your lifestyle choices or your risk factors.
- Denial, disbelief, or avoidance of your condition or your recovery.
- Grief, loss, or mourning for your previous health or your normal life.

These emotions are normal and common among people who have experienced a heart attack or heart surgery. They are part of the psychological adjustment process that occurs after a traumatic event. However, if these emotions are overwhelming, persistent, or interfere with your daily functioning, you may have a mental health condition such as post-traumatic stress disorder (PTSD), anxiety disorder, or depression. These conditions can affect your recovery and your quality of life, and they require professional help. You should talk to your doctor, a mental health counselor, or a support group if you have any signs or symptoms of these conditions.

The importance of cardiac rehabilitation and follow-up care

One of the most important steps you can take to recover from heart disease is to participate in a cardiac rehabilitation program. Cardiac rehabilitation, or cardiac rehab, is a comprehensive and personalized program that helps you improve your physical, emotional, and social well-being after a heart attack, heart failure, or other heart problems. It usually involves a team of health professionals, such as cardiologists, nurses, physiotherapists, dietitians, psychologists, and social workers, who work with you to design and monitor a plan that suits your needs and goals.

The main components of cardiac rehab are:

1. Exercise training: This involves supervised and progressive physical activity that helps you improve your cardiovascular fitness, strength, endurance, and flexibility.

Exercise training can reduce your symptoms, lower your blood pressure, improve your blood flow, and prevent further damage to your heart. It can also boost your mood, energy, and confidence. The type, intensity, duration, and frequency of exercise will depend on your condition, your risk factors, and your preferences. Your exercise program may include aerobic exercises, such as walking, cycling, or swimming, and resistance exercises, such as lifting weights or using elastic bands. You may also do stretching, balance, or relaxation exercises. You will usually start your exercise training in a hospital or a clinic, where you will be monitored by a health professional. You will then gradually transition to a home-based or community-based program, where you will exercise on your own or with a group.

2. Education and counseling: This involves learning about your condition, your treatment, your recovery, and your prevention. Education and counseling can help you understand your heart disease, its causes, its consequences, and its management. It can also help you cope with your emotions, address your fears, and overcome your barriers. You will receive information and advice on topics such as:

- The anatomy and function of your heart.

- The signs and symptoms of heart problems.

- The medications and procedures you need.

- The risk factors and complications of heart disease.

- The lifestyle changes and adjustments you need to make.

- The goals and expectations of your recovery.

- The resources and support available to you

You may receive education and counseling individually or in a group, in person or online, verbally or in writing, depending on your needs and preferences. You may also have the opportunity to ask questions, share your experiences, and learn from others who have similar conditions.

3. Behavior change and support: This involves adopting and maintaining healthy habits that can reduce your risk of future heart problems and improve your quality of life. Behavior change and support can help you modify your diet, quit smoking, manage your stress, control your weight, and adhere to your medication and treatment. You will receive guidance and encouragement from your health professionals, as well as from your family, friends, and peers. You will also learn skills and strategies to cope with challenges, overcome temptations, and sustain your motivation. You may use tools and techniques such as:

- Goal setting and action planning.
- Self-monitoring and feedback.
- Problem solving and decision making.
- Cognitive restructuring and positive thinking.
- Relaxation and mindfulness.
- Contingency management and rewards.

You may also use devices and apps that can help you track your progress, remind you of your tasks, and provide you with feedback and support.

Cardiac rehab can have many benefits for your recovery and your health. Studies have shown that cardiac rehab can:

Reduce your risk of death, heart attack, stroke, and hospitalization

- Improve your heart function, blood pressure, cholesterol, and blood sugar.

- Enhance your physical fitness, mobility, and independence.
- Alleviate your symptoms, pain, and discomfort.
- Boost your mood, self-esteem, and quality of life.
- Increase your knowledge, skills, and confidence.
- Strengthen your social support and relationships

To get the most out of cardiac rehab, you should start it as soon as possible after your heart attack or heart surgery, and continue it for at least three to six months. You should also follow the recommendations and instructions of your health professionals, and communicate with them regularly about your progress, problems, and concerns. You should also involve your family and friends in your recovery, and seek their help and support when needed.

In addition to cardiac rehab, you should also follow up with your doctor and other health professionals regularly after your heart attack or heart surgery. You should have regular check-ups, tests, and evaluations to monitor your condition, your treatment, and your recovery. You should also report any changes, difficulties, or complications that you may experience, and seek immediate medical attention if you have any signs or symptoms of a new or worsening heart problem. Your follow-up care will help you prevent or detect any problems early, and adjust or optimize your treatment if needed.

The lifestyle changes and adjustments you need to make after treatment

Another key step to recovering from heart disease is to make some lifestyle changes and adjustments that can improve your heart health and your overall well-being. These changes and adjustments may involve your diet, your smoking, your alcohol, your stress, your weight, your sleep, and your work. They may also affect your family, your friends, your hobbies, and your finances. Some of these changes and adjustments may be easy and enjoyable, while others may be hard and challenging. However, they are all important and beneficial for your recovery and your prevention.

Here are some of the lifestyle changes and adjustments you need to make after treatment:

1. Eat a heart-healthy diet: A heart-healthy diet is one that is low in saturated fat, trans fat, cholesterol, salt, and added sugar, and high in fiber, fruits, vegetables, whole grains, lean protein, and healthy fats. A heart-healthy diet can help you lower your blood pressure, cholesterol, and blood sugar, and prevent or manage obesity, diabetes, and other conditions that can increase your risk of heart disease. A heart-healthy diet can also provide you with the nutrients, energy, and satisfaction you need for your recovery and your daily activities. Some examples of heart-healthy foods are:

- Fruits, such as apples, bananas, berries, oranges, and grapes.
- Vegetables, such as broccoli, spinach, carrots, tomatoes, and peppers.
- Whole grains, such as oatmeal, brown rice, quinoa, and whole wheat bread.
- Lean protein, such as fish, poultry, eggs, beans, and nuts.
- Healthy fats, such as olive oil, avocado, flaxseed, and salmon

Some examples of foods to limit or avoid are:

- Red meat, processed meat, and organ meat.

- Butter, cream, cheese, and other full-fat dairy products.

- Margarine, shortening, and other foods that contain partially hydrogenated oils or tropical oils.

- Pastries, cakes, cookies, and other baked goods.

- Chips, crackers, popcorn, and other snacks.

- Fried foods, fast foods, and processed foods.

- Candy, chocolate, ice cream, and other sweets

To eat a heart-healthy diet, you should follow these tips:

- Plan your meals and snacks ahead of time, and shop for healthy ingredients.

- Read the nutrition labels and ingredients lists of the foods you buy, and choose the ones that are low in fat, sodium, and sugar, and high in fiber and nutrients.

- Cook your own food as much as possible, and use healthy cooking methods, such as baking, grilling, steaming, or roasting.

- Use herbs, spices, lemon juice, vinegar, or salsa to flavor your food, instead of salt, butter, or sauces.

- Control your portion sizes, and use smaller plates, bowls, and cups.

- Eat slowly, and stop when you are full.

- Drink plenty of water, and limit your intake of sugary drinks, such as soda, juice, or sports drinks.

- Limit your alcohol consumption, and avoid binge drinking.

- Treat yourself occasionally, but do not overdo it

2. Quit smoking: Smoking is one of the worst things you can do for your heart and your health. Smoking can damage your blood vessels, increase your blood pressure, reduce your oxygen supply, and make your blood more likely to clot. Smoking can also worsen your symptoms, increase your risk of complications, and delay your healing. Smoking can also harm the people around you, by exposing them to secondhand smoke. Quitting smoking can have immediate and long-term benefits for your recovery and your health. Studies have shown that quitting smoking can:

- Reduce your risk of death, heart attack, stroke, and cancer.

- Improve your blood circulation, oxygen level, and lung function.

- Lower your blood pressure, heart rate, and cholesterol.

- Ease your breathing, coughing, and wheezing.

- Enhance your taste, smell, and appearance.

- Save you money and time.

To quit smoking, you should follow these steps:

- Set a quit date, and mark it on your calendar.

- Tell your family, friends, and health professionals about your plan, and ask for their support and encouragement.

- Get rid of all your cigarettes, lighters, ashtrays, and other smoking-related items.

- Use nicotine replacement products, such as patches, gums, lozenges, or inhalers, or prescription medications, such as bupropion or varenicline, to help you cope with the withdrawal symptoms and cravings.

- Avoid triggers and temptations, such as people, places, or situations that make you want to smoke.

- Find healthy alternatives, such as chewing gum, drinking water, exercising, or calling a friend, to distract yourself from smoking.

- Reward yourself for your achievements, such as buying yourself a gift, going to a movie, or taking a trip, to celebrate your milestones.

- Seek professional help, such as a smoking cessation program, a counselor, or a hotline, if you need more guidance and support.

- Do not give up, and learn from your mistakes, if you have a slip or a relapse

3. Manage your stress: Stress is a normal and inevitable part of life, but too much stress can be harmful for your heart and your health. Stress can affect your body, your mind, and your behavior. Stress can cause your blood pressure, heart rate, and blood sugar to rise, and your blood vessels to constrict. Stress can also trigger or worsen your symptoms, such as chest pain, shortness of breath, or palpitations. Stress can also affect your mood, your thoughts, and your actions. Stress can make you feel anxious, depressed, angry, or irritable. Stress can also make you eat more, sleep less, smoke more, drink more, or exercise less. Stress can also interfere with your relationships, your work, and your hobbies. Managing your stress can help you relax, cope, and recover. Studies have shown that managing your stress can:

- Lower your blood pressure, heart rate, and blood sugar.
- Improve your blood flow and oxygen supply.
- Reduce your inflammation and oxidative stress.
- Alleviate your symptoms and pain.
- Boost your mood, self-esteem, and quality of life.
- Enhance your cognitive function, memory, and concentration.
- Improve the quality and quantity of your sleep.
- Increase your physical activity and energy level.
- Strengthen your immune system and resistance to infections

To manage your stress, you should follow these tips:

- Identify the sources and signs of your stress, and try to avoid or reduce them.

- Express your feelings and thoughts, and share your problems and concerns, with someone you trust, such as a family member, a friend, or a counselor.

- Practice relaxation techniques, such as deep breathing, meditation, yoga, tai chi, or progressive muscle relaxation, to calm your body and mind.

- Engage in enjoyable activities, such as reading, listening to music, gardening, or playing games, to distract yourself from stress and have fun.

- Maintain a positive attitude, and focus on the things you can control, change, or cope with, rather than the things you cannot.

- Set realistic and achievable goals, and prioritize and organize your tasks, to manage your time and workload.

- Seek social support, and join a group, a club, or a community, to connect with others who have similar interests, experiences, or challenges.

- Seek professional help, such as a stress management program, a therapist, or a coach, if you need more guidance and support.

- Take care of yourself, and treat yourself well, by eating well, sleeping well, exercising well, and quitting smoking and drinking.

4. Control your weight: Being overweight or obese can increase your risk of heart disease and other health problems, such as diabetes, high blood pressure, high cholesterol, and sleep apnea. Being overweight or obese can also worsen your symptoms, increase your complications, and delay your recovery. Losing weight can have many benefits for your recovery and your health. Studies have shown that losing weight can:

- Reduce your risk of death, heart attack, stroke, and heart failure.
- Improve your heart function, blood pressure, cholesterol, and blood sugar.
- Ease your symptoms, such as chest pain, shortness of breath, and fatigue.
- Enhance your physical fitness, mobility, and independence.
- Boost your mood, self-esteem, and quality of life.
- Improve your sleep quality and quantity.

- Increase your sexual function and satisfaction

To lose weight, you should follow these steps:

- Calculate your body mass index (BMI), and determine your ideal weight range, based on your height and age.
- Set a realistic and healthy weight loss goal, and monitor your progress regularly.
- Follow a balanced and low-calorie diet, and limit your intake of fat, sugar, and alcohol.
- Increase your physical activity, and burn more calories than you consume.
- Use behavioral strategies, such as self-monitoring, goal setting, feedback, and rewards, to motivate yourself and stay on track.
- Seek professional help, such as a weight management program, a dietitian, or a trainer, if you need more guidance and support.
- Do not use extreme or unsafe methods, such as fasting, skipping meals, or taking diet pills, to lose weight.

5. Improve your sleep: Sleep is essential for your heart and your health. Sleep can help you heal, restore, and rejuvenate your body and mind. Sleep can also help you regulate your hormones, blood pressure, heart rate, and blood sugar. Sleep can also affect your mood, your thoughts, and your actions. Sleep can make you feel refreshed, alert, and energetic. Sleep can also make you feel happy, calm, and optimistic. Sleep can also help you learn, remember, and perform better. Getting enough and good quality sleep can have many benefits for your recovery and your health. Studies have shown that getting enough and good quality sleep can:

- Reduce your risk of death, heart attack, stroke, and heart failure.
- Improve your heart function, blood pressure, cholesterol, and blood sugar.
- Alleviate your symptoms, such as chest pain, shortness of breath, and fatigue.
- Boost your mood, self-esteem, and quality of life.
- Enhance your cognitive function, memory, and concentration.
- Increase your physical activity and energy level.

- Strengthen your immune system and resistance to infections

To improve your sleep, you should follow these tips:

- Aim for seven to nine hours of sleep per night, and keep a regular sleep schedule.
- Create a comfortable and quiet sleeping environment, and use curtains, blinds, earplugs, or masks to block out any light or noise.
- Avoid caffeine, nicotine, alcohol, or heavy meals before bedtime, as they can interfere with your sleep quality and quantity.
- Avoid naps during the day, especially in the late afternoon or evening, as they can disrupt your sleep cycle and make it harder to fall asleep at night.
- Follow a relaxing bedtime routine, such as reading, listening to soothing music, or meditating, to unwind and prepare for sleep.
- Avoid using electronic devices, such as TV, computer, or phone, before bedtime, as they can emit blue light that can stimulate your brain and keep you awake.

- Use your bed only for sleep and sex, and not for work or other activities, and not associate it with any stress or anxiety.

- Seek professional help, such as a sleep specialist, a therapist, or a coach, if you have any sleep disorders, such as insomnia, sleep apnea, or restless legs syndrome, that may affect your sleep quality and quantity

6. Adjust your work: Work is an important and meaningful part of life, but it can also be a source of stress and strain for your heart and your health. Work can affect your recovery in various ways, depending on your type, level, and satisfaction of work. Work can provide you with income, purpose, and fulfillment. Work can also provide you with structure, routine, and social interaction. Work can also challenge you, stimulate you, and motivate you. However, work can also demand you, pressure you, and exhaust you. Work can also expose you to hazards, conflicts, and discrimination. Work can also interfere with your personal life, your leisure time, and your sleep. Adjusting your work can help you balance your recovery and your career. Adjusting your work can also help you reduce your stress and improve your performance. Adjusting your work can also help you achieve your goals and aspirations. Some of the ways you can adjust your work are:

I. Take a leave of absence, or a sick leave, from your work, if you need time to rest, heal, and recover from your heart attack or heart surgery. You should consult your doctor, your employer, and your insurance company about the duration, terms, and conditions of your leave. You should also keep in touch with your colleagues, your supervisor, and your human resources department, and update them on your progress and plans.

II. Return to work gradually, or on a part-time basis, when you feel ready and able to resume your work. You should discuss your return to work plan with your doctor, your employer, and your insurance company, and agree on the date, hours, and duties of your work. You should also communicate your needs, expectations, and concerns with your colleagues, your supervisor, and your human resources department, and seek their support and accommodation.

III. Modify your work environment, or your work conditions, to make it more comfortable and conducive for your recovery. You should request for any changes or adjustments that can help you perform your work better and safer, such as:

- Changing your workstation, or your equipment, to suit your physical abilities and limitations.

- Changing your work schedule, or your work hours, to suit your energy level and preferences.

- Changing your work location, or your work site, to reduce your travel time and expenses.

- Changing your work role, or your work responsibilities, to match your skills and interests.

- Changing your work pace, or your work load, to avoid overwork and burnout.

IV. Seek professional help, such as a vocational rehabilitation program, a counselor, or a coach, if you need more guidance and support to adjust your work. You may also consider changing your career, or your occupation, if your current work is incompatible with your recovery or your goals. You may also consider retiring from work, or quitting work, if your health, your finances, or your preferences allow you to do so.

V. Make other lifestyle changes and adjustments, as needed, to suit your recovery and your preferences. You may need to make some changes and adjustments in other aspects of your life, such as your family, your friends, your hobbies, and your finances, to cope with your condition and your treatment. These changes and adjustments may involve:

- Communicating your feelings, thoughts, and needs, and listening to those of your family and friends, to maintain and improve your relationships.

- Seeking and accepting help and support, and offering and providing help and support, to your family and friends, to share and overcome your challenges.

- Resuming and enjoying your hobbies and interests, and exploring and discovering new ones, to enrich and diversify your life.

- Managing and budgeting your finances, and planning and saving for your future, to reduce your financial stress and uncertainty.

- Making and updating your will, and arranging and organizing your affairs, to prepare for any unforeseen circumstances and events.

These lifestyle changes and adjustments may not be easy or pleasant, but they are necessary and beneficial for your recovery and your health. They can help you prevent or reduce your risk of future heart problems, and improve your quality and quantity of life. They can also help you cope with your emotions, and enhance your well-being and happiness. They can also help you achieve your personal and professional goals, and fulfill your dreams and aspirations.

The coping strategies and support resources for recovery

Recovering from heart disease can be stressful and challenging, but you do not have to do it alone. There are many coping strategies and support resources that can help you deal with your condition and your treatment, and improve your recovery and your health. These coping strategies and support resources can help you:

- Understand and accept your condition and your treatment, and cope with the changes and adjustments they entail.
- Manage and reduce your physical and emotional symptoms, pain, and discomfort.
- Learn and practice healthy habits and behaviors that can prevent or lower your risk of future heart problems.
- Overcome and resolve any problems or difficulties that may arise during your recovery.
- Enhance and maintain your physical, mental, and social well-being and happiness.

Some of the coping strategies and support resources that can help you are:

1. Self-care: Self-care is the practice of taking care of yourself, and doing things that are good for your body, mind, and soul. Self-care can help you recover from heart disease, by improving your health, alleviating your symptoms, boosting your mood, and increasing your confidence. Self-care can also help you prevent future heart problems, by reducing your risk factors, improving your resilience, and strengthening your immunity. Self-care can also help you enjoy your life, by satisfying your needs, fulfilling your desires, and expressing your personality. Some examples of self-care activities are:

- Eating a balanced and nutritious diet, and drinking plenty of water.
- Exercising regularly and moderately, and stretching and relaxing your muscles.
- Sleeping well and enough, and resting and napping when needed.
- Taking your medications and following your treatment as prescribed.
- Checking your vital signs and monitoring your condition regularly.
- Practicing good hygiene and grooming, and dressing comfortably and appropriately.
- Pampering yourself and indulging yourself occasionally, such as taking a bath, getting a massage, or buying a gift.

- Doing something creative or productive, such as writing, painting, or gardening.

- Doing something fun or entertaining, such as watching a movie, playing a game, or going to a concert.

- Doing something spiritual or meaningful, such as praying, meditating, or volunteering

2. Social support: Social support is the help and assistance that you receive from other people, such as your family, friends, neighbors, co-workers, or community members. Social support can help you recover from heart disease, by providing you with emotional, informational, instrumental, and appraisal support. Social support can also help you prevent future heart problems, by reducing your stress, improving your coping, and enhancing your relationships. Social support can also help you enjoy your life, by giving you a sense of belonging, purpose, and value. Some examples of social support activities are:

- Talking and listening to your family and friends, and sharing your feelings, thoughts, and experiences.

- Asking and offering help and advice to your family and friends, and solving your problems and concerns.

- Seeking and accepting help and assistance from your family and friends, and expressing your gratitude and appreciation.

- Spending quality time and having fun with your family and friends, and celebrating your achievements and milestones.

- Joining and participating in groups, clubs, or communities that share your interests, experiences, or challenges.

- Making and maintaining new and old friendships, and expanding your social network and circle.

- Giving and receiving compliments, feedback, and encouragement from your family, friends, and peers.

- Showing and receiving affection, love, and intimacy from your family, friends, and partner.

3. Professional help: Professional help is the guidance and support that you receive from health professionals, such as doctors, nurses, physiotherapists, dietitians, psychologists, and social workers. Professional help can help you recover from heart disease, by providing you with medical, physical, nutritional, psychological, and social services. Professional help can also help you prevent future heart problems, by providing you with education, counseling, behavior change, and follow-up care. Professional help can also help you enjoy your life, by providing you with skills, strategies, and resources that can improve your functioning and performance. Some examples of professional help activities are:

- Consulting and visiting your doctor and other health professionals regularly, and following their recommendations and instructions.
- Participating and completing a cardiac rehabilitation program, and continuing your exercise and education at home or in the community.
- Seeking and receiving mental health counseling or therapy, if you have any emotional or psychological issues, such as anxiety, depression, or PTSD.

- Seeking and receiving vocational rehabilitation or coaching, if you have any work-related issues, such as returning to work, changing your career, or retiring.

- Seeking and receiving financial counseling or planning, if you have any money-related issues, such as managing your budget, saving for your future, or making your will.

- Seeking and receiving legal counseling or representation, if you have any legal issues, such as filing a claim, suing a party, or defending a case.

- Seeking and receiving spiritual counseling or guidance, if you have any religious or existential issues, such as finding your faith, meaning, or purpose.

These coping strategies and support resources are not mutually exclusive, and they can be used together or separately, depending on your needs and preferences. You should try to use as many coping strategies and support resources as possible, and find the ones that work best for you. You should also be flexible and adaptable, and adjust your coping strategies and support resources as your recovery progresses and your situation changes.

The success stories and testimonials of heart disease survivors

Recovering from heart disease can be inspiring and rewarding, but it can also be daunting and discouraging. Sometimes, you may feel hopeful and optimistic, and other times, you may feel hopeless and pessimistic. Sometimes, you may feel proud and confident, and other times, you may feel ashamed and doubtful. Sometimes, you may feel motivated and determined, and other times, you may feel demotivated and resigned. Recovering from heart disease can be a roller coaster of emotions, and you may need some inspiration and encouragement along the way.

One of the best sources of inspiration and encouragement for your recovery is the success stories and testimonials of heart disease survivors. These are the stories and testimonials of people who have experienced a heart attack, heart failure, or other heart problems, and have recovered from them, or are recovering from them. These are the stories and testimonials of people who have faced and overcome the physical and emotional challenges of recovery, and have achieved and maintained a better quality of life. These are the stories and testimonials of people who have made and sustained the lifestyle changes and adjustments that are necessary and beneficial for recovery, and have reached and surpassed their goals and aspirations. These are the stories and testimonials of people who have learned and grown from their experience, and have found new meaning and purpose in their life.

You can find the success stories and testimonials of heart disease survivors in various places, such as:

- Books, magazines, newspapers, and websites that feature stories and interviews of heart disease survivors.

- Blogs, podcasts, videos, and social media platforms that share stories and testimonials of heart disease survivors.

- Support groups, forums, chat rooms, and online communities that connect and interact with heart disease survivors.

- Events, workshops, seminars, and conferences that invite and host heart disease survivors.

- Hospitals, clinics, and cardiac rehab centers that display and distribute stories and testimonials of heart disease survivors

You can also create and share your own success story and testimonial of recovery, and inspire and encourage others who are going through the same journey. You can write, record, or film your story and testimonial, and share it with your family, friends, health professionals, and other heart disease survivors. You can also publish, broadcast, or upload your story and testimonial, and reach a wider audience. You can also join and participate in groups, events, and programs that showcase and celebrate the success stories and testimonials of heart disease survivors.

The success stories and testimonials of heart disease survivors can have many benefits for your recovery and your health. They can:

- Provide you with information and education about your condition, your treatment, your recovery, and your prevention.

- Provide you with motivation and inspiration to overcome your challenges and achieve your goals.

- Provide you with guidance and advice to cope with your emotions and make your changes and adjustments.

- Provide you with feedback and validation to boost your confidence and self-esteem.

- Provide you with support and empathy to reduce your stress and loneliness.

- Provide you with hope and optimism to improve your mood and quality of life

To get the most out of the success stories and testimonials of heart disease survivors, you should:

- Seek and find the stories and testimonials that are relevant and relatable to your condition, your treatment, your recovery, and your goals.

- Read, listen, or watch the stories and testimonials with an open mind and a positive attitude, and learn from their experiences, insights, and lessons.

- Apply and adapt the stories and testimonials to your own situation and circumstances, and use them as examples, models, or mentors.

- Appreciate and acknowledge the stories and testimonials, and express your gratitude and admiration.

- Share and exchange the stories and testimonials with others, and create and contribute your own story and testimonial.

In summary, Recovery from heart disease is a complex process that impacts not only physical health but also emotional well-being, relationships, work, and lifestyle. Physical challenges include chest pain, shortness of breath, swelling, irregular heartbeat, infection, nausea, constipation, and sexual dysfunction. Emotional challenges include anxiety, depression, anger, guilt, and grief. These emotions are normal and can be triggered by mental health conditions like PTSD or anxiety disorder. Cardiac rehabilitation is a crucial step in recovery, involving supervised exercise training and education and counseling. Exercise training can improve cardiovascular fitness, reduce symptoms, and prevent further damage. Education and counseling can help individuals understand their condition, treatment, recovery, and prevention, and provide support for lifestyle changes and recovery goals. Individuals can receive education and counseling individually or in groups, and can learn from others with similar conditions.

Cardiac rehab is a crucial step in recovery from heart disease, aiming to reduce the risk of future heart problems and improve quality of life. It involves adopting healthy habits, such as diet modification, quitting smoking, managing stress, controlling weight, and adhering to medication and treatment. It can improve heart function, physical fitness, and independence. To maximize benefits, it is recommended to start cardiac rehab as soon as possible after a heart attack or surgery and continue for at least three to six months. Regular follow-ups with health professionals and family members are also essential.

After treatment, lifestyle changes and adjustments, such as a heart-healthy diet, should be made. These changes should include a balanced diet low in saturated fat, trans fat, cholesterol, salt, and added sugar, and a focus on healthy fats and fruits. Limiting or avoiding certain foods can also help in recovery.

Quit smoking is crucial for heart health as it damages blood vessels, increases blood pressure, and reduces oxygen supply. Quitting smoking can reduce the risk of death, heart attack, stroke, and cancer, improve blood circulation, lower blood pressure, and improve lung function. To manage stress, identify sources and reduce stress, express feelings, practice relaxation techniques, engage in enjoyable activities, maintain a positive attitude, set realistic goals, seek social support, and seek professional help. Controlling weight can also help reduce the risk of heart disease, improve heart function, ease symptoms, enhance physical fitness, and improve mood, self-esteem, and quality of life. Losing weight can also improve physical fitness, mobility, and independence, boost mood, self-esteem, and quality of life, and increase sexual function and satisfaction.

To lose weight, calculate your BMI, set a realistic weight loss goal, follow a balanced diet, increase physical activity, use behavioral strategies, seek professional help, and avoid extreme methods. Improve your sleep by aiming for seven to nine hours of sleep per night, creating a comfortable environment, avoiding caffeine, nicotine, alcohol, or heavy meals before bedtime, avoiding naps during the day, following a relaxing bedtime routine, and using electronic devices before bedtime. Seek professional help if you have sleep disorders.

Adjust your work to balance your recovery and career. Take a leave of absence, return to work gradually, modify your work environment, or consider changing your career or occupation. Seek professional help if needed, and make lifestyle changes to suit your recovery and preferences. Adjusting your work can help reduce stress, improve performance, and help achieve your goals.

Heart disease recovery requires lifestyle changes and adjustments in various aspects of life, such as communication, seeking support, and managing finances. These changes can help prevent future heart problems, improve quality of life, and enhance emotional well-being. Coping strategies and support resources can help manage physical and emotional symptoms, learn healthy habits, overcome difficulties, and maintain well-being. Self-care activities include eating a balanced diet, exercising regularly, sleeping well, taking medications, maintaining good hygiene, and engaging in creative activities. Social support from family, friends, and community members can provide emotional, informational, instrumental, and appraisal support, reducing stress, improving coping, and enhancing relationships. These activities can help you enjoy life, achieve personal and professional goals, and fulfill your dreams and aspirations.

Professional help from health professionals can help recover from heart disease by providing medical, physical, psychological, and social services. It can also help prevent future heart problems by providing education, counseling, behavior change, and follow-up care. Coping strategies and support resources can be used together or separately, depending on individual needs. Success stories and testimonials of heart disease survivors can provide inspiration and encouragement for recovery. These stories can be found in various places, such as books, blogs, social media, support groups, events, and clinics. Sharing your own success story and testimonial can inspire others and reach a wider audience. Being flexible and adaptable is essential as recovery progresses.

Heart disease survivors' success stories and testimonials can provide valuable information, motivation, guidance, feedback, support, and hope for recovery and health. To benefit from these stories, individuals should seek relatable ones, apply them to their own situation, appreciate them, and share them with others. Recovery from heart disease is a complex process that affects physical, emotional, and social well-being. Physical challenges include chest pain, shortness of breath, swelling, irregular heartbeat, infection, nausea, constipation, and sexual dysfunction. Emotional challenges include anxiety, fear, depression, anger, guilt, denial, and grief.

Cardiac rehabilitation is a crucial step in recovery, involving supervised exercise training and education and counseling. This program helps improve cardiovascular fitness, strength, endurance, and flexibility, reducing symptoms, lowering blood pressure, and preventing further damage. It can also help individuals understand their condition, treatment, recovery, and prevention. It is essential to consult a doctor, mental health counselor, or support group for any signs or symptoms of these conditions.

Chapter 3: Lifestyle

Heart disease is a serious and common condition that affects millions of people around the world. It can cause chest pain, shortness of breath, irregular heartbeat, and even death. Heart disease can be caused by many factors, such as genetics, age, smoking, high blood pressure, high cholesterol, diabetes, obesity, and stress. However, heart disease can also be prevented and managed by adopting a healthy lifestyle that includes a balanced diet and regular exercise. In this chapter, we will explore the role of diet and nutrition, the recommended foods and supplements, the practical and delicious recipes and meal plans, the role of exercise and physical activity, and the suitable and enjoyable exercises and activities for your heart health.

The Role of Diet and Nutrition

Diet and nutrition play a crucial role in preventing and managing heart disease. What you eat and drink can affect your blood pressure, cholesterol, blood sugar, inflammation, and weight, which are all risk factors for heart disease. A healthy diet can help lower your risk of heart disease by:

1. Reducing the amount of saturated fat, trans fat, salt, and added sugar in your diet. These can raise your blood pressure, cholesterol, and triglycerides, which can damage your arteries and increase your risk of heart attack and stroke. Instead, choose foods that are low in fat, salt, and sugar, such as fruits, vegetables, whole grains, lean proteins, and low-fat dairy products.

2. Increasing the amount of fiber in your diet. Fiber can help lower your cholesterol, blood sugar, and blood pressure, as well as make you feel full and prevent overeating. Fiber can also help lower inflammation, which can contribute to heart disease. Aim for at least 25 grams of fiber per day from sources such as fruits, vegetables, beans, nuts, seeds, and whole grains.

3. Including more omega-3 fatty acids in your diet. Omega-3 fatty acids are a type of unsaturated fat that can help lower your triglycerides, blood pressure, and inflammation, as well as improve your heart rhythm and blood flow. Omega-3 fatty acids are found in fatty fish,

such as salmon, tuna, mackerel, herring, and sardines, as well as in flaxseeds, chia seeds, walnuts, and soybeans. Aim for at least two servings of fatty fish per week, or take a fish oil supplement if you don't eat fish.

4. Adding more antioxidants and phytochemicals to your diet. Antioxidants and phytochemicals are compounds that can help protect your cells from oxidative stress and inflammation, which can damage your arteries and lead to heart disease. Antioxidants and phytochemicals are found in colorful fruits and vegetables, such as berries, citrus fruits, tomatoes, carrots, spinach, kale, broccoli, and cabbage, as well as in tea, coffee, cocoa, spices, and herbs. Aim for at least five servings of fruits and vegetables per day, and enjoy a variety of colors and flavors.

5. Drinking enough water and limiting alcohol. Water is essential for your body to function properly and to flush out toxins and waste. Water can also help regulate your body temperature, blood pressure, and blood volume, which can affect your heart health. Aim for at least eight glasses of water per day, or more if you exercise or live in a hot climate. Alcohol, on the other hand, can raise your blood

pressure, triglycerides, and calories, which can increase your risk of heart disease. Alcohol can also interfere with your medications and affect your heart rhythm. If you drink alcohol, limit yourself to no more than one drink per day for women and two drinks per day for men, and avoid binge drinking.

The Recommended Foods and Supplements

To follow a heart-healthy diet, you need to know which foods and supplements are good for your heart and which ones are not. Here are some of the recommended foods and supplements for your heart health:

1. Fruits and vegetables: Fruits and vegetables are rich in fiber, antioxidants, phytochemicals, vitamins, and minerals, which can help lower your risk of heart disease. They can also help you control your weight, blood pressure, cholesterol, and blood sugar. Choose fresh, frozen, or canned fruits and vegetables, and avoid those with added salt, sugar, or sauces. Eat a variety of colors and types, and aim for at least five servings per day.

2. Whole grains: Whole grains are grains that have not been refined or processed, and they contain the entire grain kernel, including the bran, germ, and endosperm. Whole grains are high in fiber, vitamins, minerals, and phytochemicals, which can help lower your cholesterol, blood pressure, blood sugar, and inflammation. They can also help you feel full and prevent overeating. Choose whole grains, such as oatmeal, brown rice, quinoa, barley, buckwheat, and whole wheat bread, pasta, and cereal, and avoid refined grains, such as white bread, white rice, and white flour products. Aim for at least three servings of whole grains per day.

3. Lean proteins: Lean proteins are proteins that are low in fat and calories, and they provide essential amino acids, which are the building blocks of your muscles, organs, and tissues. Lean proteins can help you maintain your muscle mass, metabolism, and immune system, as well as lower your cholesterol and blood pressure. They can also help you feel full and prevent overeating. Choose lean proteins, such as skinless chicken, turkey, fish, eggs, tofu, beans, lentils, and low-fat dairy products, and avoid fatty meats, such as bacon, sausage, ham, and ribs. Aim for at least two servings of lean proteins per day, and vary your sources.

4. Healthy fats: Healthy fats are fats that are unsaturated, meaning they have one or more double bonds in their chemical structure. Healthy fats can help lower your cholesterol, triglycerides, and inflammation, as well as improve your heart rhythm and blood flow. They can also help you absorb fat-soluble vitamins, such as A, D, E, and K, and provide energy and satiety. Choose healthy fats, such as olive oil, canola oil, avocado, nuts, seeds, and fatty fish, and avoid unhealthy fats, such as butter, lard, margarine, shortening, and coconut oil. Aim for no more than 25 to 35 percent of your total calories from fat, and limit your saturated fat intake to less than 10 percent and your trans fat intake to zero.

5. **Supplements**: Supplements are products that contain vitamins, minerals, herbs, or other substances that are intended to supplement your diet and provide additional health benefits. Supplements can help fill in the gaps in your nutrition, especially if you have a deficiency or a medical condition that affects your absorption or

metabolism of nutrients. However, supplements are not a substitute for a balanced diet, and they can also have side effects, interactions, and contraindications. Therefore, you should always consult your doctor before taking any supplements, and follow the dosage and instructions on the label. Some of the supplements that may be beneficial for your heart health include:

- **Fish oil**: Fish oil contains omega-3 fatty acids, which can help lower your triglycerides, blood pressure, and inflammation, as well as improve your heart rhythm and blood flow. Fish oil can also help prevent or treat conditions such as arrhythmia, angina, heart failure, and stroke. The American Heart Association recommends that people with coronary artery disease take 1 gram of omega-3 fatty acids per day, and that people with high triglycerides take 2 to 4 grams per day. However, fish oil can also cause bleeding, bruising, and allergic reactions, and it can interact with blood thinners, blood pressure medications, and diabetes medications. Therefore, you should always consult your doctor before taking fish oil, and monitor your blood tests regularly.

- **Coenzyme Q10**: Coenzyme Q10, or CoQ10, is a substance that is naturally produced by your body and is involved in the production of energy in your cells. CoQ10 can help protect your heart from oxidative stress and inflammation, as well as improve your heart function and blood pressure. CoQ10 can also help prevent or treat conditions such as heart failure, angina, and hypertension. The typical dose of CoQ10 is 100 to 200 milligrams per day, but it can vary depending on your age, weight, and health status. However, CoQ10 can also cause nausea, diarrhea, headache, and insomnia, and it can interact with blood thinners, blood pressure medications, and statins. Therefore, you should always consult your doctor before taking CoQ10, and monitor your blood tests regularly.

- **Magnesium**: Magnesium is a mineral that is essential for many functions in your body, such as muscle contraction, nerve transmission, bone formation, and enzyme activity. Magnesium can help lower your blood pressure, regulate your heart rhythm, and prevent or treat conditions such as arrhythmia, angina, and heart failure. The recommended dietary allowance of magnesium for adults is 310 to 420 milligrams per day, depending on your age and gender. However, magnesium can also cause diarrhea, cramps, nausea, and vomiting, and it can interact with antibiotics, diuretics, and bisphosphonates. Therefore, you should always consult your doctor before taking magnesium, and monitor your blood tests regularly.

The Practical and Delicious Recipes and Meal Plans

Eating a heart-healthy diet does not have to be boring or bland. You can enjoy a variety of delicious and satisfying dishes that are good for your heart and your taste buds. In this section, we will provide some practical and easy recipes and meal plans that you can follow or adapt to your preferences and needs. These recipes and meal plans are based on the principles of the Mediterranean diet, which is one of the most studied and recommended diets for heart health. The Mediterranean diet emphasizes fruits, vegetables, whole grains, beans, nuts, seeds, olive oil, fish, poultry, herbs, spices, and moderate amounts of dairy, eggs, and wine. The Mediterranean diet is low in red meat, processed meat, refined grains, added sugar, and saturated fat, and high in fiber, antioxidants, phytochemicals, and healthy fats. The Mediterranean diet has been shown to lower the risk of heart disease, stroke, diabetes, obesity, and cognitive decline, as well as improve the quality of life and longevity.

Here are some examples of recipes and meal plans that you can try or modify:

<u>Breakfast</u>

1. Oatmeal with fresh or dried fruits, nuts, seeds, and cinnamon. You can cook the oatmeal with water, milk, or plant-based milk, and sweeten it with honey, maple syrup, or stevia. You can also add some protein powder, flaxseeds, chia seeds, or hemp seeds for extra nutrition and satiety.

2. Greek yogurt with granola, berries, and honey. You can choose low-fat or full-fat yogurt, depending on your preference and calorie needs. You can also make your own

granola with oats, nuts, seeds, coconut, and maple syrup, and bake it in the oven until golden and crunchy.

3. Whole wheat toast with avocado, egg, and tomato. You can mash the avocado with some lemon juice, salt, and pepper, and spread it on the toast. You can cook the egg to your liking, such as scrambled, fried, or poached, and place it on top of the avocado. You can slice the tomato and add it to the sandwich, or serve it on the side with some olive oil and basil.

4. Smoothie with banana, spinach, almond milk, peanut butter, and cocoa powder. You can blend all the ingredients together until smooth and creamy, and enjoy it as a drink or a bowl. You can also add some ice, vanilla extract, or protein powder for extra flavor and nutrition.

Lunch

1. Salad with mixed greens, cherry tomatoes, cucumber, olives, feta cheese, and grilled chicken. You can toss the salad with some olive oil, lemon juice, salt, pepper, and oregano, or use your favorite dressing. You can also substitute the chicken with tuna, salmon, or beans for more protein options.

2. Sandwich with whole wheat bread, hummus, roasted vegetables, and cheese. You can spread the hummus on the bread, and layer it with roasted vegetables, such as eggplant, zucchini, bell pepper, onion, and mushroom. You can also add some cheese, such as mozzarella, cheddar, or goat cheese, and melt it in the oven or microwave. You can also serve the sandwich with some salad, soup, or fruit for a complete meal.

3. Pasta with whole wheat or chickpea noodles, tomato sauce, and meatballs. You can cook the pasta according to the package directions, and drain it. You can make the tomato sauce with canned or fresh tomatoes, garlic, onion, basil, and salt, and simmer it until thick and fragrant. You can make the meatballs with lean ground beef, turkey, or chicken, bread crumbs, egg, parsley, salt, and pepper, and bake them in the oven or cook them in the skillet. You can combine the pasta, sauce, and meatballs, and sprinkle some parmesan cheese on top.

4. Rice bowl with brown rice, black beans, corn, salsa, and avocado. You can cook the rice according to the package directions, and fluff it with a fork. You can heat the beans

and corn in a saucepan or microwave, and season them with some cumin, chili powder, and salt. You can chop the avocado and toss it with some lime juice, salt, and cilantro. You can assemble the bowl with the rice, beans, corn, salsa, and avocado, and enjoy it hot or cold.

<u>Dinner</u>

1. Salmon with roasted potatoes and asparagus. You can season the salmon with some salt, pepper, garlic, and lemon, and bake it in the oven until flaky and tender. You can cut the potatoes into wedges and toss them with some olive oil, rosemary, salt, and pepper, and roast them in the oven until golden and crispy. You can trim the asparagus and drizzle some olive oil, salt, and pepper, and roast them in the oven until crisp and tender.

2. Chicken and vegetable stir-fry with brown rice or quinoa. You can cut the chicken into bite-sized pieces and marinate it with some soy sauce, honey, garlic, ginger, and cornstarch. You can chop the vegetables, such as broccoli, carrot, bell pepper, onion, and mushroom, and stir-fry them in a wok or skillet with some oil, salt, and pepper. You can cook the chicken in the same wok or skillet until cooked

through, and add some more soy sauce, honey, vinegar, and sesame oil for the sauce. You can serve the stir-fry with brown rice or quinoa, and garnish it with some sesame seeds and scallions.

3. Vegetable and bean soup with whole wheat bread. You can sauté some onion, garlic, celery, and carrot in a large pot with some oil, salt, and pepper. You can add some vegetable broth, water, bay leaf, thyme, and rosemary, and bring it to a boil. You can add some beans, such as kidney, cannellini, or black beans, and simmer the soup until the beans are soft. You can also add some spinach, kale, or cabbage at the end for some extra greens. You can serve the soup with some whole wheat bread, and sprinkle some parmesan cheese on top.

4. Pizza with whole wheat or cauliflower crust, tomato sauce, cheese, and toppings. You can make the crust with whole wheat flour, yeast, water, oil, salt, and sugar, and knead it until smooth and elastic. You can also make the crust with cauliflower, egg, cheese, and seasonings, and press it into a baking sheet. You can bake the crust in the oven until firm and golden. You can spread the tomato

sauce on the crust, and sprinkle some cheese, such as mozzarella, cheddar, or feta. You can also add some toppings, such as pepperoni, ham, chicken, mushrooms, olives, pineapple, or spinach. You can bake the pizza in the oven until the cheese is melted and bubbly. You can cut the pizza into slices and enjoy it hot or cold.

The Role of Exercise and Physical Activity

Exercise and physical activity are also important for preventing and managing heart disease. Exercise and physical activity can help you:

- Strengthen your heart muscle and improve your blood circulation. This can lower your resting heart rate and blood pressure, and reduce your risk of heart attack and stroke.

- Burn calories and fat, and maintain a healthy weight. This can lower your cholesterol, triglycerides, and blood sugar, and prevent or treat conditions such as obesity, diabetes, and metabolic syndrome.

- Reduce stress and improve your mood. This can lower your cortisol and adrenaline levels, and increase your endorphins and serotonin levels. This can also help you cope with anxiety, depression, and anger, which can affect your heart health.

- Enhance your immune system and prevent infections. This can lower your inflammation and oxidative stress, and protect your arteries and cells from damage.

- Improve your sleep quality and duration. This can help you rest and recover, and regulate your hormones and metabolism.

The American Heart Association recommends that adults get at least 150 minutes of moderate-intensity aerobic exercise, or 75 minutes of vigorous-intensity aerobic exercise, or a combination of both, per week. Aerobic exercise is any activity that increases your heart rate and breathing, such as walking, jogging, cycling, swimming, dancing, or playing sports. You should also do some muscle-strengthening exercises, such as lifting weights, doing push-ups, or using resistance bands, at least two times per week. Muscle-strengthening exercises can help you build and maintain your muscle mass, bone density, and metabolism, as well as improve your posture and balance.

However, before you start any exercise program, you should always consult your doctor, especially if you have any heart condition, such as coronary artery disease, heart failure, arrhythmia, or valve disease. Your doctor can help you determine the best type, intensity, frequency, and duration of exercise for your specific condition and goals. You should also monitor your heart rate, blood pressure, and symptoms, such as chest pain, shortness of breath, dizziness, or palpitations, during and after exercise. If you experience any of these symptoms, you should stop exercising and seek medical attention immediately.

The Suitable and Enjoyable Exercises and Activities

To follow a heart-healthy exercise program, you need to find the suitable and enjoyable exercises and activities that match your fitness level, preferences, and needs. Here are some of the suitable and enjoyable exercises and activities for your heart health:

1. **Walking**: Walking is one of the simplest and most accessible forms of exercise. It can help you improve your cardiovascular fitness, burn calories, and reduce stress. You can walk anywhere, anytime, and at your own pace. You can also vary your speed, distance, and terrain, to challenge yourself and avoid boredom. You can walk alone, with a partner, or with a group, to make it more fun and social. You can also use a pedometer, a smartphone app, or a fitness tracker, to measure your steps, distance, and calories burned, and set goals and track your progress. Aim for at least 10,000 steps per day, or 30 minutes of brisk walking, most days of the week.

2. **Jogging**: Jogging is a form of running that is slower and less intense than sprinting. It can help you improve your aerobic endurance, burn more calories and fat, and strengthen your muscles and bones. You can jog on a treadmill, a track, a road, or a trail, depending on your preference and availability. You can also vary your speed, distance, and interval, to challenge yourself and avoid boredom. You can jog alone, with a partner, or with a group, to make it more fun and social. You can also use a stopwatch, a smartphone app, or a fitness tracker, to

measure your time, distance, and calories burned, and set goals and track your progress. Aim for at least 20 minutes of jogging, three times per week, or more if you can.

3. **Cycling**: Cycling is a form of exercise that involves riding a bicycle. It can help you improve your cardiovascular fitness, burn calories and fat, and strengthen your muscles and joints. You can cycle on a stationary bike, a road bike, or a mountain bike, depending on your preference and availability. You can also vary your speed, distance, and resistance, to challenge yourself and avoid boredom. You can cycle alone, with a partner, or with a group, to make it more fun and social. You can also use a speedometer, a smartphone app, or a fitness tracker, to measure your speed, distance, and calories burned, and set goals and track your progress. Aim for at least 30 minutes of cycling, three times per week, or more if you can.

4. **Swimming**: Swimming is a form of exercise that involves moving through water. It can help you improve your cardiovascular fitness, burn calories and fat, and strengthen your muscles and lungs. Swimming is also a low-impact exercise, which means it does not put much

stress on your joints and bones, and it is suitable for people with arthritis, injuries, or disabilities. You can swim in a pool, a lake, or an ocean, depending on your preference and availability. You can also vary your stroke, speed, and distance, to challenge yourself and avoid boredom. You can swim alone, with a partner, or with a group, to make it more fun and social. You can also use a stopwatch, a smartphone app, or a fitness tracker, to measure your time, distance, and calories burned, and set goals and track your progress. Aim for at least 20 minutes of swimming, three times per week, or more if you can.

5. **Dancing**: Dancing is a form of exercise that involves moving your body to music. It can help you improve your cardiovascular fitness, burn calories and fat, and strengthen your muscles and coordination. Dancing is also a fun and creative exercise, which can boost your mood and self-esteem. You can dance to any music, style, and tempo, depending on your preference and mood. You can dance alone, with a partner, or with a group, to make it more fun and social. You can also use a music player, a smartphone app, or a fitness tracker, to measure your time, steps, and calories burned, and set goals and track your progress. Aim

for at least 30 minutes of dancing, three times per week, or more if you can.

These arc some of the examples of exercises and activities that you can do for your heart health. However, you can also choose any other exercise or activity that you like and enjoy, as long as it is safe and appropriate for your condition and goals. The most important thing is to be consistent and regular, and to have fun and feel good. Remember, exercise is not only good for your heart, but also for your mind, body, and soul.

Keeping a healthy weight reduces the burden on the heart and lowers the risk of heart disease, as well as other health issues like diabetes.

Chapter 4: Prevention

Heart disease is the leading cause of death worldwide, claiming more than 17 million lives each year. It is a complex and multifactorial condition that involves various risk factors, such as genetics, age, gender, ethnicity, lifestyle, and environment. However, many of these risk factors are modifiable, meaning that they can be changed or controlled by adopting healthy habits and behaviors. In fact, according to the World Health Organization, at least 80% of premature deaths from heart disease and stroke could be prevented by addressing the main risk factors: tobacco use, unhealthy diet, physical inactivity, and harmful use of alcohol.

In this chapter, we will explore the key habits and behaviors that can prevent or reduce the risk of heart disease, as well as the effective and proven ways to quit smoking, lower blood pressure, and control cholesterol. We will also discuss the stress management and relaxation techniques that can protect your heart, and the importance of regular check-ups and screenings for heart disease.

Finally, we will look at the future trends and innovations in heart disease prevention, such as personalized medicine, digital health, and gene therapy.

The Key Habits and Behaviors that Can Prevent or Reduce the Risk of Heart Disease

The most important thing you can do to prevent or reduce the risk of heart disease is to adopt a healthy lifestyle. A healthy lifestyle consists of four main components: a balanced diet, regular physical activity, moderate alcohol consumption, and no smoking. These habits and behaviors can help you maintain a healthy weight, lower your blood pressure, improve your blood lipids, reduce inflammation, and prevent or delay the development of atherosclerosis, the buildup of fatty deposits in the arteries that can lead to heart attack or stroke.

A Balanced Diet

A balanced diet is one that provides adequate amounts of nutrients, such as carbohydrates, proteins, fats, vitamins, minerals, and fiber, while limiting the intake of salt, sugar, saturated fat, trans fat, and cholesterol. A balanced diet can help you prevent or manage various risk factors for heart disease, such as obesity, diabetes, hypertension, and dyslipidemia.

There is no single diet that is best for everyone, as different people have different needs and preferences. However, some general principles that can guide you to a healthy eating pattern are:

- Eat more fruits, vegetables, whole grains, legumes, nuts, seeds, and fish. These foods are rich in antioxidants, phytochemicals, fiber, omega-3 fatty acids, and other beneficial nutrients that can lower your risk of heart disease.

- Eat less red meat, processed meat, refined grains, sweets, and sugary drinks. These foods are high in calories, sodium, sugar, saturated fat, trans fat, and cholesterol, which can increase your risk of heart disease.

- Choose healthy fats over unhealthy fats. Healthy fats, such as monounsaturated and polyunsaturated fats, are found in olive oil, canola oil, sunflower oil, avocado, nuts, seeds, and fish. These fats can lower your LDL (bad) cholesterol and raise your HDL (good) cholesterol, as well as reduce inflammation and oxidative stress. Unhealthy fats, such as saturated and trans fats, are found in butter, lard, coconut oil, palm oil, margarine, shortening, baked goods, fried foods, and processed foods. These fats can raise your LDL cholesterol and lower your HDL cholesterol, as well as increase inflammation and oxidative stress.

- Limit your salt intake to less than 5 grams per day. Salt, or sodium chloride, is essential for maintaining fluid balance, nerve function, and muscle contraction. However, too much salt can raise your blood pressure, which can damage your arteries and increase your risk of heart disease. Most of the salt we consume comes from processed foods, such as bread, cheese, canned foods, sauces, snacks, and fast foods. Therefore, it is important to read the nutrition labels and choose low-sodium or sodium-free products, as well as to avoid adding salt to your food or using salty condiments, such as soy sauce, ketchup, and mustard.

- Limit your sugar intake to less than 10% of your total energy intake. Sugar, or sucrose, is a simple carbohydrate that provides energy for the body. However, too much sugar can lead to weight gain, diabetes, tooth decay, and increased triglycerides, which can raise your risk of heart disease. Most of the sugar we consume comes from added sugars, such as table sugar, honey, syrups, and molasses, as well as from sugary drinks, such as soda, juice, and sports drinks. Therefore, it is important to limit your consumption of these products, as well as to choose natural or artificial sweeteners, such as stevia, xylitol, or aspartame, instead of sugar.

A balanced diet can be achieved by following various dietary patterns, such as the Mediterranean diet, the DASH diet, the vegetarian diet, or the flexitarian diet. These diets have been shown to lower the risk of heart disease and other chronic diseases, as well as to improve the quality of life. However, the most important thing is to find a diet that suits your needs, preferences, and culture, and to stick to it consistently.

Regular Physical Activity

Regular physical activity is any bodily movement that requires energy expenditure, such as walking, jogging, cycling, swimming, dancing, gardening, or playing sports. Regular physical activity can help you prevent or reduce the risk of heart disease by:

- Improving your cardiovascular fitness, which means your heart and lungs can deliver more oxygen and nutrients to your muscles and organs.

- Strengthening your heart muscle, which means your heart can pump more blood with less effort.

- Lowering your blood pressure, which means your arteries are less likely to be damaged by high pressure.

- Improving your blood lipids, which means your LDL cholesterol is lower and your HDL cholesterol is higher.

- Reducing your body fat, which means your weight is within a healthy range and your risk of obesity, diabetes, and metabolic syndrome is lower.

- Enhancing your insulin sensitivity, which means your blood sugar is more stable and your risk of diabetes is lower.

- Reducing your inflammation, which means your immune system is less likely to attack your own tissues and cause damage to your arteries.

- Boosting your mood, which means your stress level is lower and your mental health is better.

The World Health Organization recommends that adults aged 18 to 64 years should do at least 150 minutes of moderate-intensity aerobic physical activity, or 75 minutes of vigorous-intensity aerobic physical activity, or an equivalent combination of both, per week. Moderate-intensity physical activity is any activity that makes you breathe faster and feel warmer, such as brisk walking, cycling, or swimming. Vigorous-intensity physical activity is any activity that makes you breathe hard and fast, such as running, jumping, or playing soccer. Aerobic physical activity is any activity that uses large muscle groups and increases your heart rate, such as walking, jogging, cycling, swimming, or dancing.

In addition to aerobic physical activity, the World Health Organization also recommends that adults should do muscle-strengthening activities involving major muscle groups, such as the legs, hips, back, abdomen, chest, shoulders, and arms, at least twice a week. Muscle-strengthening activities are any activities that make your muscles work harder than usual, such as lifting weights, doing push-ups, or using resistance bands. Muscle-strengthening activities can help you increase your muscle mass, strength, and endurance, as well as prevent or delay the loss of muscle and bone that occurs with aging.

Regular physical activity can be achieved by incorporating it into your daily routine, such as taking the stairs instead of the elevator, walking or cycling to work or school, or doing household chores. You can also join a gym, a sports club, or a fitness class, or find a workout buddy, to make physical activity more fun and social. However, the most important thing is to find a physical activity that you enjoy, that is safe and appropriate for your level of fitness, and that you can do regularly and consistently.

Moderate Alcohol Consumption

Alcohol is a psychoactive substance that affects the brain and the body in various ways. Alcohol can have both beneficial and harmful effects on the heart, depending on the amount and frequency of consumption. Moderate alcohol consumption is defined as up to one drink per day for women and up to two drinks per day for men. One drink is equivalent to 12 grams of pure alcohol, which is found in 10 ounces of beer, 5 ounces of wine, or 1.5 ounces of liquor. Moderate alcohol consumption can help you prevent or reduce the risk of heart disease by:

- Increasing your HDL cholesterol, which can help remove excess LDL cholesterol from your arteries.
- Reducing your blood clotting, which can lower your risk of heart attack or stroke caused by a blood clot in your arteries.
- Relaxing your blood vessels, which can lower your blood pressure and improve your blood flow.
- Reducing your stress, which can lower your cortisol level and improve your mental health.

However, excessive alcohol consumption, which is more than the moderate amount, can have the opposite effects and increase your risk of heart disease by:

- Increasing your LDL cholesterol, which can clog your arteries and lead to atherosclerosis.
- Increasing your blood pressure, which can damage your arteries and strain your heart.
- Increasing your triglycerides, which can contribute to the formation of fatty deposits in your arteries.
- Increasing your inflammation, which can trigger an immune response that can damage your arteries and heart.
- Increasing your risk of arrhythmia, which is an abnormal heartbeat that can cause your heart to beat too fast, too slow, or irregularly.
- Increasing your risk of cardiomyopathy, which is a weakening of the heart muscle that can impair its ability to pump blood.
- Increasing your risk of heart failure, which is a condition where your heart cannot meet the demand of your body for blood and oxygen.

- Increasing your risk of stroke, which is a sudden interruption of blood flow to the brain that can cause brain damage or death.

Therefore, it is important to drink alcohol in moderation, or not at all, if you have a history of heart disease, high blood pressure, high cholesterol, diabetes, or liver disease. You should also avoid binge drinking, which is defined as consuming more than four drinks for men or three drinks for women in a single occasion. Binge drinking can cause a sudden spike in your blood pressure, heart rate, and blood alcohol level, which can increase your risk of heart attack, stroke, or sudden cardiac death.

No Smoking

Smoking is one of the most harmful habits for your heart, as well as for your lungs, skin, teeth, and overall health. Smoking can increase your risk of heart disease by:

- Increasing your blood pressure, which can damage your arteries and strain your heart.
- Increasing your heart rate, which can make your heart work harder and consume more oxygen.

- Decreasing your oxygen level, which can deprive your heart and other organs of the oxygen they need to function properly.

- Increasing your carbon monoxide level, which can bind to your hemoglobin and reduce its ability to carry oxygen to your tissues.

- Increasing your blood clotting, which can block your arteries and cause a heart attack or stroke.

- Increasing your inflammation, which can trigger an immune response that can damage your arteries and heart.

- Increasing your oxidative stress, which can cause cellular damage and accelerate the aging process.

- Damaging your endothelium, which is the inner lining of your arteries that helps regulate blood flow and prevent atherosclerosis.

- Reducing your HDL cholesterol, which can impair your ability to remove excess LDL cholesterol from your arteries.

- Increasing your risk of arrhythmia, which is an abnormal heartbeat that can cause your heart to beat too fast, too slow, or irregularly.

- Increasing your risk of coronary artery spasm, which is a sudden narrowing of the arteries that supply blood to your heart, which can cause chest pain or a heart attack.
- Increasing your risk of sudden cardiac death, which is an unexpected death due to a heart problem that occurs within an hour of the onset of symptoms.

Therefore, it is essential to quit smoking, or never start, if you want to prevent or reduce the risk of heart disease. Quitting smoking can have immediate and long-term benefits for your heart, such as:

- Lowering your blood pressure and heart rate within minutes.
- Improving your blood circulation and oxygen level within hours.
- Reducing your carbon monoxide level and increasing your hemoglobin level within a day.
- Reducing your risk of heart attack and stroke within weeks.
- Improving your lung function and exercise capacity within months.

- Reducing your inflammation and oxidative stress within a year.

- Repairing your endothelium and increasing your HDL cholesterol within a few years.

- Reducing your risk of heart disease and death by half within five years.

Quitting smoking can be challenging, but it is not impossible. There are various methods and resources that can help you quit, such as nicotine replacement therapy, medication, counseling, support groups, apps, and websites. The most important thing is to find a method that works for you, and to seek help from your doctor, family, friends, or other smokers who have successfully quit. You should also prepare yourself for the withdrawal symptoms, such as cravings, irritability, anxiety, depression, insomnia, weight gain, and difficulty concentrating, that may occur when you stop smoking. These symptoms are temporary and will subside over time, as your body adjusts to being nicotine-free. You should also avoid triggers, such as stress, alcohol, coffee, or other smokers, that may tempt you to smoke again. You should also reward yourself for your progress, such as by saving the money you would have spent on cigarettes, or by treating yourself to something you enjoy. Quitting smoking is one of the best decisions you can make for your heart and your health. It is never too late to quit, and the benefits are worth the effort.

The Effective and Proven Ways to Quit Smoking, Lower Blood Pressure, and Control Cholesterol

As we have seen in the previous section, smoking, high blood pressure, and high cholesterol are three of the major risk factors for heart disease. Therefore, it is crucial to quit smoking, lower blood pressure, and control cholesterol, if you want to prevent or reduce the risk of heart disease. In this section, we will explore the effective and proven ways to achieve these goals, as well as the benefits and challenges of each method.

Quitting Smoking

Quitting smoking is one of the most effective and proven ways to prevent or reduce the risk of heart disease, as well as to improve your overall health and well-being. However, quitting smoking can also be one of the most difficult and challenging tasks, as nicotine, the addictive substance in tobacco, can create a strong physical and psychological dependence. Therefore, quitting smoking requires a combination of motivation, determination, and support, as well as the use of appropriate methods and resources.

There are various methods and resources that can help you quit smoking, such as:

1. Nicotine replacement therapy (NRT): This is a method that provides you with a low dose of nicotine, without the harmful chemicals in tobacco smoke, to help you cope with the withdrawal symptoms and cravings. NRT can come in different forms, such as patches, gums, lozenges, inhalers, or sprays, and can be obtained over-the-counter or by prescription. NRT can double your chances of quitting successfully, but you should follow the instructions carefully and consult your doctor before using it, especially if you have a history of heart disease, high blood pressure, diabetes, or other medical conditions.

2. **Medication**: This is a method that involves taking prescription drugs, such as bupropion or varenicline, that can help you quit smoking by reducing your nicotine dependence, withdrawal symptoms, and cravings.

Medication can also double your chances of quitting successfully, but you should consult your doctor before using it, as it may have side effects or interactions with other drugs or conditions. You should also follow the dosage and duration of treatment as prescribed by your doctor, and not stop taking the medication abruptly or without medical advice.

3. **Counseling**: This is a method that involves talking to a trained professional, such as a doctor, nurse, therapist, or counselor, who can provide you with advice, guidance, support, and feedback on your quitting process. Counseling can help you identify your reasons for quitting, your triggers for smoking, your coping strategies, and your progress and challenges. Counseling can also help you deal with the emotional and psychological aspects of quitting, such as stress, anxiety, depression, or low self-esteem. Counseling can be done individually or in a group, in person or by phone, online or offline, and can be combined with other methods, such as NRT or medication. Counseling can increase your chances of quitting successfully by up to 50%, but you should find a counselor

who is qualified, experienced, and trustworthy, and who can meet your needs and preferences.

4. Support groups: This is a method that involves joining a group of people who are also trying to quit smoking, or who have already quit, and who can provide you with mutual support, encouragement, and advice. Support groups can help you share your experiences, challenges, and successes, as well as learn from others' tips, strategies, and stories. Support groups can also help you feel less alone, isolated, or judged, and more motivated, confident, and accountable. Support groups can be found in your community, workplace, or online, and can be combined with other methods, such as counseling, NRT, or medication. Support groups can increase your chances of quitting successfully by up to 50%, but you should find a group that is suitable, accessible, and compatible with your personality and goals.

5. Apps and websites: This is a method that involves using digital tools, such as apps or websites, that can help you quit smoking by providing you with information, tips, feedback, reminders, rewards, and other features. Apps and websites can help you track your smoking habits, set your quit date, monitor your progress, calculate your savings, access your support network, and access other resources, such as NRT, medication, counseling, or support groups. Apps and websites can be used on your smartphone, tablet, or computer, and can be customized to your needs and preferences. Apps and websites can increase your chances of quitting successfully by up to 50%, but you should find a tool that is reliable, user-friendly, and effective, and that does not compromise your privacy or security.

These are some of the most common and popular methods and resources that can help you quit smoking, but there are also other methods and resources that may work for you, such as hypnosis, acupuncture, herbal remedies, or e-cigarettes. However, you should be careful and cautious about these methods and resources, as they may not be scientifically proven, regulated, or safe, and they may have adverse effects on your health or your quitting process. Therefore, you should always consult your doctor before trying any of these methods and resources, and do your own research and evaluation.

The best method and resource for quitting smoking is the one that works for you, and that you can stick to until you are smoke-free. You may need to try different methods and resources, or combine them, to find the most effective and suitable one for you. You may also need to adjust your method and resource as you go along, depending on your progress and challenges. However, the most important thing is to have a clear and strong motivation for quitting, and to seek and accept help and support from others, such as your doctor, family, friends, or other quitters.

Quitting smoking is not easy, but it is possible. Millions of people have successfully quit smoking, and so can you. You just need to take the first step, and keep going until you reach your goal. Quitting smoking will not only benefit your heart, but also your lungs, skin, teeth, and overall health and well-being. Quitting smoking will also benefit your family, friends, and society, as you will reduce your exposure to secondhand smoke, and save money and resources. Quitting smoking will also benefit your future, as you will increase your life expectancy, quality of life, and happiness. Quitting smoking is one of the best decisions you can make for yourself and your heart. It is never too late to quit, and the benefits are worth the effort. You can do it.

Lowering Blood Pressure

Lowering blood pressure is another effective and proven way to prevent or reduce the risk of heart disease, as well as to improve your overall health and well-being. However, lowering blood pressure can also be challenging, as high blood pressure, or hypertension, is often a silent and chronic condition that may not cause any symptoms or signs until it is too late. Therefore, lowering blood pressure requires regular monitoring, treatment, and lifestyle changes.

There are various methods and resources that can help you lower your blood pressure, such as:

1. **Medication**: This is a method that involves taking prescription drugs, such as diuretics, beta-blockers, calcium channel blockers, angiotensin-converting enzyme inhibitors, angiotensin receptor blockers, or others, that can help you lower your blood pressure by relaxing your blood vessels, reducing your blood volume, slowing down your heart rate, or blocking certain hormones. Medication can be

very effective in lowering your blood pressure, but you should consult your doctor before using it, as it may have side effects or interactions with other drugs or conditions. You should also follow the dosage and duration of treatment as prescribed by your doctor, and not stop taking the medication abruptly or without medical advice.

2. **Diet**: This is a method that involves eating a balanced and healthy diet, as described in the previous section, that can help you lower your blood pressure by providing adequate amounts of nutrients, while limiting the intake of salt, sugar, saturated fat, trans fat, and cholesterol. A specific dietary pattern that has been shown to lower blood pressure is the DASH diet, which stands for Dietary Approaches to Stop Hypertension. The DASH diet emphasizes fruits, vegetables, whole grains, low-fat dairy products, lean meats, nuts, seeds, and legumes, while limiting sodium, sweets, and red meats. The DASH diet can lower your blood pressure by up to 14 mmHg, which is comparable to the effect of some medications, but you should consult your doctor before starting it, as it may not be suitable for everyone, especially if you have kidney disease or other medical conditions.

3. **Physical activity**: This is a method that involves doing regular physical activity, as described in the previous section, that can help you lower your blood pressure by improving your cardiovascular fitness, strengthening your heart muscle, lowering your body fat, enhancing your insulin sensitivity, reducing your inflammation, and boosting your mood. The World Health Organization recommends that adults aged 18 to 64 years should do at least 150 minutes of moderate-intensity aerobic physical activity, or 75 minutes of vigorous-intensity aerobic physical activity, or an equivalent combination of both, per week, as well as muscle-strengthening activities involving major muscle groups, at least twice a week. Physical activity can lower your blood pressure by up to 10 mmHg, which is comparable to the effect of some medications, but you should consult your doctor before starting it, especially if you have a history of heart disease, high blood pressure, or other medical conditions.

4. **Stress management**: This is a method that involves coping with stress, which is a normal and inevitable part of life, but which can also raise your blood pressure, by affecting your nervous system, hormones, and blood

vessels. Stress management can help you lower your blood pressure by relaxing your mind and body, and reducing your cortisol level and inflammation. There are various stress management techniques that can help you cope with stress, such as:

- Breathing exercises: These are exercises that involve inhaling and exhaling deeply and slowly, which can help you calm your nervous system, lower your heart rate, and relax your blood vessels. Breathing exercises can be done anytime and anywhere, and can be combined with other techniques, such as meditation, yoga, or tai chi.
- Meditation: This is a technique that involves focusing your attention on a single object, such as your breath, a word, a sound, or an image, which can help you clear your mind, reduce your negative thoughts, and enhance your awareness and mindfulness. Meditation can be done in a quiet and comfortable place, and can be combined with other techniques, such as breathing exercises, yoga, or tai chi.

- <u>Yoga</u>: This is a technique that involves performing a series of physical poses, movements, and stretches, which can help you improve your flexibility, balance, strength, and posture. Yoga can also help you calm your mind, reduce your stress, and enhance your well-being. Yoga can be done in a class, at home, or online, and can be combined with other techniques, such as breathing exercises, meditation, or tai chi.

- <u>Tai chi</u>: This is a technique that involves performing a series of slow and graceful movements, which can help you improve your coordination, agility, and stability. Tai chi can also help you calm your mind, reduce your stress, and enhance your well-being. Tai chi can be done in a class, at home, or online, and can be combined with other techniques, such as breathing exercises, meditation, or yoga.

- <u>Biofeedback</u>: This is a technique that involves using a device, such as a monitor, a sensor, or an app, that can measure and display your physiological signals, such as your heart rate, blood pressure, skin temperature, or muscle tension, which can help you become aware of your body's response to stress, and learn how to control it. Biofeedback can be done with the help of a trained professional, or by yourself, and can be combined with other techniques, such as breathing exercises, meditation, yoga, or tai chi.

5. **Cognitive behavioral therapy (CBT)**: This is a technique that involves talking to a trained professional, such as a therapist or a counselor, who can help you identify and change your negative thoughts, beliefs, and behaviors, that can cause or worsen your stress, and replace them with positive ones. CBT can help you cope with stress, anxiety, depression, or other psychological problems, that can affect your blood pressure. CBT can be done individually or in a group, in person or by phone, online or offline, and can be combined with other techniques, such as medication, diet, or physical activity.

These are some of the most common and popular stress management techniques that can help you lower your blood pressure, but there are also other techniques that may work for you, such as listening to music, reading a book, watching a movie, playing a game, gardening, or spending time with your family, friends, or pets. However, you should be careful and cautious about some techniques, such as smoking, drinking, eating, or shopping, that may seem to relieve your stress, but that may actually increase your blood pressure or have other negative effects on your health or your quitting process. Therefore, you should always consult your doctor before trying any of these techniques, and do your own research and evaluation.

The best method and resource for lowering your blood pressure is the one that works for you, and that you can stick to until you reach your goal. You may need to try different methods and resources, or combine them, to find the most effective and suitable one for you. You may also need to adjust your method and resource as you go along, depending on your progress and challenges. However, the most important thing is to monitor your blood pressure regularly, and to seek and accept help and support from others, such as your doctor, family, friends, or other people with high blood pressure.

Lowering your blood pressure is not easy, but it is possible. Millions of people have successfully lowered their blood pressure, and so can you. You just need to take the first step, and keep going until you reach your goal. Lowering your blood pressure will not only benefit your heart, but also your brain, kidneys, eyes, and overall health and well-being. Lowering your blood pressure will also benefit your family, friends, and society, as you will reduce your risk of heart attack, stroke, or other complications, and save money and resources. Lowering your blood pressure will also benefit your future, as you will increase your life expectancy, quality of life, and happiness.

Controlling Cholesterol

Controlling cholesterol is another effective and proven way to prevent or reduce the risk of heart disease, as well as to improve your overall health and well-being. However, controlling cholesterol can also be challenging, as high cholesterol, or hypercholesterolemia, is often a silent and chronic condition that may not cause any symptoms or signs until it is too late. Therefore, controlling cholesterol requires regular monitoring, treatment, and lifestyle changes.

There are various methods and resources that can help you control your cholesterol, such as:

1. **Medication**: This is a method that involves taking prescription drugs, such as statins, fibrates, bile acid sequestrants, niacin, or others, that can help you lower your cholesterol by reducing its production, absorption, or reabsorption in the liver, intestine, or bloodstream. Medication can be very effective in lowering your cholesterol, but you should consult your doctor before using it, as it may have side effects or interactions with other drugs or conditions. You should also follow the dosage and duration of treatment as prescribed by your doctor, and not stop taking the medication abruptly or without medical advice.

2. **Diet**: This is a method that involves eating a balanced and healthy diet, as described in the previous section, that can help you lower your cholesterol by providing adequate amounts of nutrients, while limiting the intake of salt, sugar, saturated fat, trans fat, and cholesterol. A specific

dietary pattern that has been shown to lower cholesterol is the TLC diet, which stands for Therapeutic Lifestyle Changes. The TLC diet emphasizes fruits, vegetables, whole grains, low-fat dairy products, lean meats, fish, nuts, seeds, and legumes, while limiting sodium, sweets, and red meats. The TLC diet can lower your cholesterol by up to 15%, but you should consult your doctor before starting it, as it may not be suitable for everyone, especially if you have diabetes or other medical conditions.

3. **Physical activity:** This is a method that involves doing regular physical activity, as described in the previous section, that can help you lower your cholesterol by improving your cardiovascular fitness, strengthening your heart muscle, lowering your body fat, enhancing your insulin sensitivity, reducing your inflammation, and boosting your mood. The World Health Organization recommends that adults aged 18 to 64 years should do at least 150 minutes of moderate-intensity aerobic physical activity, or 75 minutes of vigorous-intensity aerobic physical activity, or an equivalent combination of both, per week, as well as muscle-strengthening activities involving major muscle groups, at least twice a week. Physical

activity can lower your cholesterol by up to 10%, but you should consult your doctor before starting it, especially if you have a history of heart disease, high blood pressure, or other medical conditions.

4. **Supplements**: This is a method that involves taking natural or synthetic substances, such as omega-3 fatty acids, plant sterols, soluble fiber, garlic, or others, that can help you lower your cholesterol by providing beneficial nutrients, or by interfering with its production, absorption, or reabsorption in the liver, intestine, or bloodstream. Supplements can be obtained over-the-counter or by prescription, and can be taken in the form of pills, capsules, liquids, powders, or foods. Supplements can lower your cholesterol by up to 10%, but you should consult your doctor before using them, as they may have side effects or interactions with other drugs or conditions. You should also follow the dosage and duration of use as recommended by your doctor or the manufacturer, and not exceed the safe or effective amount.

These are some of the most common and popular methods and resources that can help you control your cholesterol, but there are also other methods and resources that may work for you, such as red yeast rice, soy, green tea, or others. However, you should be careful and cautious about these methods and resources, as they may not be scientifically proven, regulated, or safe, and they may have adverse effects on your health or your quitting process. Therefore, you should always consult your doctor before trying any of these methods and resources, and do your own research and evaluation.

The best method and resource for controlling your cholesterol is the one that works for you, and that you can stick to until you reach your goal. You may need to try different methods and resources, or combine them, to find the most effective and suitable one for you. You may also need to adjust your method and resource as you go along, depending on your progress and challenges. However, the most important thing is to monitor your cholesterol regularly, and to seek and accept help and support from others, such as your doctor, family, friends, or other people with high cholesterol.

Controlling your cholesterol is not easy, but it is possible. Millions of people have successfully controlled their cholesterol, and so can you. You just need to take the first step, and keep going until you reach your goal. Controlling your cholesterol will not only benefit your heart, but also your brain, liver, gallbladder, and overall health and well-being. Controlling your cholesterol will also benefit your family, friends, and society, as you will reduce your risk of heart attack, stroke, or other complications, and save money and resources. Controlling your cholesterol will also benefit your future, as you will increase your life expectancy, quality of life, and happiness.

The Stress Management and Relaxation Techniques that Can Protect Your Heart

Stress is a normal and inevitable part of life, that can have both positive and negative effects on your heart. Stress can be positive, when it motivates you to perform better, achieve your goals, or overcome challenges. Stress can also be negative, when it overwhelms you, exceeds your coping capacity, or persists for a long time. Negative stress can harm your heart, by affecting your nervous system, hormones, and blood vessels, as well as your behavior, emotions, and thoughts.

Negative stress can affect your heart in various ways, such as:

- Raising your blood pressure, which can damage your arteries and strain your heart.
- Increasing your heart rate, which can make your heart work harder and consume more oxygen.
- Decreasing your oxygen level, which can deprive your heart and other organs of the oxygen they need to function properly.
- Increasing your blood clotting, which can block your arteries and cause a heart attack or stroke.
- Increasing your inflammation, which can trigger an immune response that can damage your arteries and heart.
- Increasing your oxidative stress, which can cause cellular damage and accelerate the aging process.
- Damaging your endothelium, which is the inner lining of your arteries that helps regulate blood flow and prevent atherosclerosis.

- Reducing your HDL cholesterol, which can impair your ability to remove excess LDL cholesterol from your arteries.

- Increasing your risk of arrhythmia, which is an abnormal heartbeat that can cause your heart to beat too fast, too slow, or irregularly.

- Increasing your risk of coronary artery spasm, which is a sudden narrowing of the arteries that supply blood to your heart, which can cause chest pain or a heart attack.

- Increasing your risk of sudden cardiac death, which is an unexpected death due to a heart problem that occurs within an hour of the onset of symptoms.

Therefore, it is important to manage your stress, and to practice relaxation techniques, that can protect your heart, as well as your overall health and well-being. Stress management and relaxation techniques can help you cope with stress, by relaxing your mind and body, and reducing your cortisol level and inflammation. There are various stress management and relaxation techniques that can help you protect your heart, such as:

1. Breathing exercises: These are exercises that involve inhaling and exhaling deeply and slowly, which can help you calm your nervous system, lower your heart rate, and relax your blood vessels. Breathing exercises can be done anytime and anywhere, and can be combined with other techniques, such as meditation, yoga, or tai chi.

2. **Meditation**: This is a technique that involves focusing your attention on a single object, such as your breath, a word, a sound, or an image, which can help you clear your mind, reduce your negative thoughts, and enhance your awareness and mindfulness. Meditation can be done in a quiet and comfortable place, and can be combined with other techniques, such as breathing exercises, yoga, or tai chi.

3. **Yoga**: This is a technique that involves performing a series of physical poses, movements, and stretches, which can help you improve your flexibility, balance, strength, and posture. Yoga can also help you calm your mind, reduce your stress, and enhance your well-being. Yoga can be done in a class, at home, or online, and can be combined

with other techniques, such as breathing exercises, meditation, or tai chi.

4. Tai chi: This is a technique that involves performing a series of slow and graceful movements, which can help you improve your coordination, agility, and stability. Tai chi can also help you calm your mind, reduce your stress, and enhance your well-being. Tai chi can be done in a class, at home, or online, and can be combined with other techniques, such as breathing exercises, meditation, or yoga.

5. Biofeedback: This is a technique that involves using a device, such as a monitor, a sensor, or an app, that can measure and display your physiological signals, such as your heart rate, blood pressure, skin temperature, or muscle tension, which can help you become aware of your body's response to stress, and learn how to control it. Biofeedback can be done with the help of a trained professional, or by yourself, and can be combined with other techniques, such as breathing exercises, meditation, yoga, or tai chi.

6. Cognitive behavioral therapy (CBT): This is a technique that involves talking to a trained professional, such as a therapist or a counselor, who can help you identify and change your negative thoughts, beliefs, and behaviors, that can cause or worsen your stress, and replace them with positive ones. CBT can help you cope with stress, anxiety, depression, or other psychological problems, that can affect your blood pressure. CBT can be done individually or in a group, in person or by phone, online or offline, and can be combined with other techniques, such as medication, diet, or physical activity.

These are some of the most common and popular stress management and relaxation techniques that can help you protect your heart, but there are also other techniques that may work for you, such as listening to music, reading a book, watching a movie, playing a game, gardening, or spending time with your family, friends, or pets. However, you should be careful and cautious about some techniques, such as smoking, drinking, eating, or shopping, that may seem to relieve your stress, but that may actually increase your blood pressure or have other negative effects on your health or your quitting process. Therefore, you should always consult your doctor before trying any of these techniques, and do your own research and evaluation.

The best method and resource for managing your stress and practicing relaxation is the one that works for you, and that you can stick to until you reach your goal. You may need to try different methods and resources, or combine them, to find the most effective and suitable one for you. You may also need to adjust your method and resource as you go along, depending on your progress and challenges. However, the most important thing is to recognize your stress, and to seek and accept help and support from others, such as your doctor, family, friends, or other people who are stressed.

Managing your stress and practicing relaxation is not easy, but it is possible. Millions of people have successfully managed their stress and practiced relaxation, and so can you. You just need to take the first step, and keep going until you reach your goal. Managing your stress and practicing relaxation will not only benefit your heart, but also your mind, body, and soul. Managing your stress and practicing relaxation will also benefit your family, friends, and society, as you will reduce your risk of heart disease and other complications, and save money and resources. Managing your stress and practicing relaxation will also benefit your future, as you will increase your life expectancy, quality of life, and happiness.

The Importance of Regular Check-ups and Screenings for Heart Disease

Regular check-ups and screenings for heart disease are another way to prevent or reduce the risk of heart disease, as well as to improve your overall health and well-being. Regular check-ups and screenings for heart disease can help you detect and diagnose any heart problems early, before they become serious or life-threatening. Regular check-ups and screenings for heart disease can also help you monitor and manage your risk factors, such as blood pressure, cholesterol, blood sugar, weight, and smoking. Regular check-ups and screenings for heart disease can also help you evaluate and improve your treatment and lifestyle, such as medication, diet, physical activity, stress management, and relaxation.

There are various types of check-ups and screenings for heart disease that you can do, such as:

1. Physical examination: This is a check-up that involves a general assessment of your health, such as your medical history, family history, symptoms, signs, and risk factors. A physical examination can help you identify any potential or existing heart problems, such as chest pain, shortness of breath, palpitations, or edema. A physical examination can also help you measure your vital signs, such as your blood pressure, heart rate, temperature, and oxygen saturation. A physical examination can be done by your doctor, nurse, or other health care provider, and should be done at least once a year, or more often if you have a history of heart disease, high blood pressure, high cholesterol, diabetes, or other medical conditions.

2. Blood tests: These are tests that involve taking a sample of your blood, usually from your arm, and analyzing it in a laboratory. Blood tests can help you measure your blood levels of various substances, such as cholesterol, triglycerides, glucose, hemoglobin, and others, that can indicate your risk of heart disease. Blood tests can also help you diagnose or rule out certain heart conditions, such as anemia, infection, inflammation, or heart failure. Blood tests can be done by your doctor, nurse, or other health care provider, and should be done at least once a year, or more often if you have a history of heart disease, high blood pressure, high cholesterol, diabetes, or other medical conditions.

3. Electrocardiogram (ECG or EKG): This is a test that involves attaching electrodes to your chest, arms, and legs, and recording the electrical activity of your heart. An ECG can help you measure your heart rate, rhythm, and conduction, and detect any abnormalities, such as arrhythmia, ischemia, infarction, or hypertrophy. An ECG can also help you diagnose or rule out certain heart conditions, such as angina, heart attack, or heart failure. An ECG can be done by your doctor, nurse, or other health care provider, and should be done at least once a year, or more often if you have a history of heart disease, high blood pressure, high cholesterol, diabetes, or other medical conditions.

4. Echocardiogram: This is a test that involves using an ultrasound device to create images of your heart. An echocardiogram can help you measure your heart size, shape, structure, function, and blood flow, and detect any abnormalities, such as valve problems, wall motion abnormalities, or chamber enlargement. An echocardiogram can also help you diagnose or rule out certain heart conditions, such as heart failure, cardiomyopathy, or congenital heart defects. An echocardiogram can be done by your doctor, nurse, or other health care provider, and should be done at least once a year, or more often if you have a history of heart disease, high blood pressure, high cholesterol, diabetes, or other medical conditions.

5. Stress test: This is a test that involves exercising on a treadmill, bike, or other device, while your heart rate, blood pressure, ECG, and oxygen level are monitored. A stress test can help you measure your heart's response to physical exertion, and detect any signs of reduced blood flow or oxygen supply to your heart. A stress test can also help you diagnose or rule out certain heart conditions, such as coronary artery disease, angina, or heart attack. A stress test can be done by your doctor, nurse, or other health care provider, and should be done at least once a year, or more often if you have a history of heart disease, high blood pressure, high cholesterol, diabetes, or other medical conditions.

6. Coronary angiogram: This is a test that involves inserting a thin tube, called a catheter, into an artery in your groin, arm, or neck, and advancing it to your heart. A dye is then injected through the catheter, and X-ray images are taken to show the blood flow and blockages in your coronary arteries. A coronary angiogram can help you measure the degree and location of any narrowing or obstruction in your coronary arteries, and determine the best treatment option, such as medication, angioplasty, or bypass surgery. A coronary angiogram can also help you diagnose or rule out certain heart conditions, such as coronary artery disease, angina, or heart attack. A coronary angiogram can be done by your doctor, nurse, or other health care provider, and should be done only if you have symptoms or signs of heart disease, or if other tests are inconclusive or abnormal.

These are some of the most common and important check-ups and screenings for heart disease that you can do, but there are also other tests that may be done, depending on your symptoms, signs, risk factors, and medical conditions. However, you should always consult your doctor before doing any of these tests, and follow their recommendations and instructions. You should also understand the purpose, procedure, benefits, risks, and results of each test, and ask any questions or concerns that you may have.

Regular check-ups and screenings for heart disease can help you prevent or reduce the risk of heart disease, as well as to improve your overall health and well-being. Regular check-ups and screenings for heart disease can also help you detect and diagnose any heart problems early, before they become serious or life-threatening. Regular check-ups and screenings for heart disease can also help you monitor and manage your risk factors, such as blood pressure, cholesterol, blood sugar, weight, and smoking. Regular check-ups and screenings for heart disease can also help you evaluate and improve your treatment and lifestyle, such as medication, diet, physical activity, stress management, and relaxation.

The Future Trends and Innovations in Heart Disease Prevention

Heart disease prevention is a dynamic and evolving field, that is influenced by the advances in science, technology, and medicine, that are constantly creating new opportunities and challenges for the prevention of heart disease. In this section, we will explore some of the future trends and innovations in heart disease prevention, such as personalized medicine, digital health, and gene therapy.

Personalized Medicine

Personalized medicine is an approach that involves tailoring the prevention, diagnosis, and treatment of heart disease to the individual characteristics, needs, and preferences of each patient. Personalized medicine can help improve the effectiveness, safety, and efficiency of heart disease prevention, by taking into account the genetic, molecular, environmental, and behavioral factors that influence the risk and response of each patient.

Personalized medicine can be achieved by using various tools and technologies, such as:

1. **Genomics**: This is the study of the genome, which is the complete set of DNA, or genetic material, of an organism. Genomics can help identify the genetic variations, such as single nucleotide polymorphisms (SNPs), that can affect the risk and response of each patient to heart disease and its prevention. Genomics can also help develop new drugs, biomarkers, and diagnostic tests, that can target the specific genes or pathways involved in heart disease and its prevention.

2. **Proteomics**: This is the study of the proteome, which is the complete set of proteins, or functional molecules, of an organism. Proteomics can help measure the levels and activities of the proteins that can affect the risk and response of each patient to heart disease and its prevention. Proteomics can also help discover new drugs, biomarkers, and diagnostic tests, that can target the specific proteins or pathways involved in heart disease and its prevention.

3. **Metabolomics**: This is the study of the metabolome, which is the complete set of metabolites, or small molecules, of an organism. Metabolomics can help analyze the metabolic profiles, or chemical fingerprints, of the

tissues, fluids, or excretions of each patient, that can reflect the risk and response of each patient to heart disease and its prevention. Metabolomics can also help identify new drugs, biomarkers, and diagnostic tests, that can target the specific metabolites or pathways involved in heart disease and its prevention.

4. **Pharmacogenomics**: This is the study of how the genes of each patient affect the response to drugs, such as their efficacy, safety, and dosage. Pharmacogenomics can help predict the optimal drug and dose for each patient, based on their genetic profile, and avoid adverse drug reactions, drug interactions, or drug resistance. Pharmacogenomics can also help develop new drugs, that can target the specific genes or pathways involved in heart disease and its prevention.

Personalized medicine can offer many benefits for the prevention of heart disease, such as:

- Improving the accuracy and reliability of the diagnosis and prognosis of heart disease, by using more precise and sensitive tests and biomarkers, that can detect the presence, severity, and progression of heart disease, and the risk of complications, in each patient.

- Enhancing the effectiveness and safety of the treatment and prevention of heart disease, by using more specific and targeted drugs and interventions, that can modulate the genes, proteins, or metabolites involved in heart disease, and avoid or minimize the side effects, toxicity, or resistance, in each patient.

- Increasing the efficiency and cost-effectiveness of the health care system, by reducing the trial and error, waste, and duplication, of the conventional one-size-fits-all approach, and by optimizing the allocation and utilization of the resources, based on the needs and preferences of each patient.

- Empowering the patients and improving their quality of life, by providing them with more information, options, and control, over their health and well-being, and by involving them in the decision-making and management of their heart disease and its prevention.

Personalized medicine can also pose some challenges and limitations for the prevention of heart disease, such as:

- Increasing the complexity and uncertainty of the diagnosis and prognosis of heart disease, by generating large amounts of data, that may be difficult to interpret, integrate, and validate, and that may vary depending on the time, place, and condition, of each patient.

- Raising the ethical, legal, and social issues of the treatment and prevention of heart disease, by creating new dilemmas, such as the privacy, security, and ownership, of the genetic and personal information, the access, affordability, and availability, of the personalized drugs and interventions, and the responsibility, liability, and accountability, of the health care providers and stakeholders.

- Requiring the collaboration and coordination of the health care system, by demanding the development and implementation of new standards, regulations, and policies, that can ensure the quality, safety, and efficacy, of the personalized medicine, and the education, training, and communication, of the health care professionals and patients, that can enable the adoption and integration, of the personalized medicine.

Personalized medicine is a promising and exciting trend and innovation in heart disease prevention, that can revolutionize the way we prevent, diagnose, and treat heart disease, and improve the health and well-being of each patient. However, personalized medicine is also a complex and challenging field, that requires more research, development, and evaluation, to overcome the barriers and limitations, and to realize the full potential and benefits, of personalized medicine.

Digital Health

Digital health is an approach that involves using information and communication technologies, such as computers, smartphones, wearables, sensors, or others, to collect, store, analyze, and share health-related data, that can help improve the prevention, diagnosis, and treatment of heart disease. Digital health can help enhance the accessibility, availability, and affordability of health care, by enabling the remote, real-time, and personalized delivery and management of health care, and by empowering the patients and improving their engagement and satisfaction.

Digital health can be achieved by using various tools and technologies, such as:

1. Electronic health records (EHRs): These are digital versions of the medical records, that can store and display the health information, such as the medical history, symptoms, signs, tests, treatments, and outcomes, of each patient. EHRs can help improve the quality and safety of health care, by facilitating the access, exchange, and integration, of the health information, among the health care providers and stakeholders, and by reducing the errors, delays, and costs, of the paper-based records.

2. Telemedicine: This is the delivery of health care services, such as consultation, diagnosis, treatment, or monitoring, through the use of telecommunication technologies, such as phone, video, or internet, that can connect the health care providers and patients, who are separated by distance, time, or location. Telemedicine can help improve the accessibility and availability of health care, by overcoming the barriers, such as the distance, travel, or transportation, that may prevent the patients from receiving the health care services, and by providing the health care services, to the underserved, rural, or remote, populations.

3. Mobile health (mHealth): This is the delivery of health care services, through the use of mobile devices, such as smartphones, tablets, or wearables, that can collect, store, analyze, and share, the health-related data, such as the vital signs, symptoms, behaviors, or outcomes, of each patient. mHealth can help improve the affordability and personalization of health care, by reducing the costs, and increasing the convenience, of the health care services, and by providing the health care services, that are tailored to the needs and preferences, of each patient.

4. Artificial intelligence (AI): This is the simulation of human intelligence, by machines, such as computers, software, or robots, that can perform tasks, such as learning, reasoning, or problem-solving, that require human intelligence. AI can help improve the effectiveness and efficiency of health care, by augmenting the capabilities, and supporting the decisions, of the health care providers and patients, and by automating the tasks, and optimizing the processes, of the health care system.

Digital health can offer many benefits for the prevention of heart disease, such as:

1. Improving the accuracy and reliability of the diagnosis and prognosis of heart disease, by using more advanced and sophisticated tools and technologies, that can collect, store, analyze, and share, large amounts of data, that can detect the presence, severity, and progression, of heart disease, and the risk of complications, in each patient.

2. Enhancing the effectiveness and safety of the treatment and prevention of heart disease, by using more specific and targeted tools and technologies, that can deliver and manage, the appropriate drugs and interventions, that can modulate the risk factors and outcomes, of heart disease, and avoid or minimize the side effects, toxicity, or resistance, in each patient.

3. Increasing the efficiency and cost-effectiveness of the health care system, by using more innovative and

disruptive tools and technologies, that can reduce the waste and duplication, of the conventional health care system, and by optimizing the allocation and utilization, of the resources, based on the demand and supply, of the health care services.

4. Empowering the patients and improving their quality of life, by using more interactive and engaging tools and technologies, that can provide them with more information, options, and control, over their health and well-being, and by involving them in the decision-making and management, of their heart disease and its prevention.

Digital health can also pose some challenges and limitations for the prevention of heart disease, such as:

1. Increasing the complexity and uncertainty of the diagnosis and prognosis of heart disease, by generating large amounts of data, that may be difficult to interpret, integrate, and validate, and that may vary depending on the source, quality, and reliability, of the data.

2. Raising the ethical, legal, and social issues of the treatment and prevention of heart disease, by creating new dilemmas, such as the privacy, security, and ownership, of

the data, the access, affordability, and availability, of the digital tools and technologies, and the responsibility, liability, and accountability, of the health care providers and stakeholders.

3. Requiring the collaboration and coordination of the health care system, by demanding the development and implementation of new standards, regulations, and policies, that can ensure the quality, safety, and efficacy, of the digital health, and the education, training, and communication, of the health care professionals and patients, that can enable the adoption and integration, of the digital health.

Digital health is a promising and exciting trend and innovation in heart disease prevention, that can transform the way we prevent, diagnose, and treat heart disease, and improve the health and well-being of each patient. However, digital health is also a complex and challenging field, that requires more research, development, and evaluation, to overcome the barriers and limitations, and to realize the full potential and benefits, of digital health.

Gene Therapy

Gene therapy is an approach that involves modifying or replacing the genes, or the units of heredity, of an organism, that can affect the risk and response of heart disease and its prevention. Gene therapy can help correct or compensate for the genetic defects or variations, that can cause or contribute to heart disease, or enhance or introduce new genes or functions, that can prevent or treat heart disease.

Gene therapy can be achieved by using various tools and technologies, such as:

1. **Vectors**: These are vehicles, such as viruses, plasmids, or nanoparticles, that can carry and deliver the genes of interest, to the target cells or tissues, of the organism. Vectors can help transfer the genes of interest, either by integrating them into the genome, or by expressing them transiently, of the target cells or tissues, and by avoiding or minimizing the immune response, or the rejection, of the organism.

2. **Gene editing**: This is a technique, such as CRISPR-Cas9, ZFNs, or TALENs, that can alter or modify the genes of interest, by adding, deleting, or replacing,

specific sequences of DNA, in the genome, of the target cells or tissues, of the organism. Gene editing can help correct or compensate for the genetic defects or variations, that can cause or contribute to heart disease, or enhance or introduce new genes or functions, that can prevent or treat heart disease.

3. Gene regulation: This is a technique, such as RNA interference, antisense oligonucleotides, or epigenetic modification, that can control or influence the expression or activity, of the genes of interest, by interfering, blocking, or modifying, the transcription, translation, or function, of the genes, in the target cells or tissues, of the organism. Gene regulation can help reduce or increase the expression or activity, of the genes of interest, that can cause or contribute to heart disease, or prevent or treat heart disease.

Gene therapy can offer many benefits for the prevention of heart disease, such as:

- Improving the accuracy and reliability of the diagnosis and prognosis of heart disease, by using more precise and sensitive tools and technologies, that can identify and characterize the genetic defects or variations, that can affect the risk and response of heart disease and its prevention, in each patient.

- Enhancing the effectiveness and safety of the treatment and prevention of heart disease, by using more specific and targeted tools and technologies, that can correct or compensate for the genetic defects or variations, that can cause or contribute to heart disease, or enhance or introduce new genes or functions, that can prevent or treat heart disease, in each patient.

- Increasing the efficiency and cost-effectiveness of the health care system, by using more innovative and disruptive tools and technologies, that can provide a permanent or long-lasting solution, for the genetic causes or contributors, of heart disease, and by reducing the need or dependence, on the conventional drugs and interventions, for the prevention and treatment, of heart disease.

- Empowering the patients and improving their quality of life, by using more personalized and customized tools and technologies, that can address the individual genetic characteristics, needs, and preferences, of each patient, and by involving them in the decision-making and management, of their heart disease and its prevention.

Gene therapy can also pose some challenges and limitations for the prevention of heart disease, such as:

- Increasing the complexity and uncertainty of the diagnosis and prognosis of heart disease, by generating large amounts of data, that may be difficult to interpret, integrate, and validate, and that may vary depending on the type, source, and quality, of the genes, vectors, and tools, used for the gene therapy.
- Raising the ethical, legal, and social issues of the treatment and prevention of heart disease, by creating new dilemmas, such as the safety, efficacy, and regulation, of the gene therapy, the consent, autonomy, and rights, of the patients, and the implications, consequences, and responsibilities, of the genetic modification, of the organism.
- Requiring the collaboration and coordination of the health care system, by demanding the development

and implementation of new standards, regulations, and policies, that can ensure the quality, safety, and efficacy, of the gene therapy, and the education, training, and communication, of the health care professionals and patients, that can enable the adoption and integration, of the gene therapy.

Gene therapy is a promising and exciting trend and innovation in heart disease prevention, that can revolutionize the way we prevent, diagnose, and treat heart disease, and improve the health and well-being of each patient. However, gene therapy is also a complex and challenging field, that requires more research, development, and evaluation, to overcome the barriers and limitations, and to realize the full potential and benefits, of gene therapy.

Heart disease prevention is a vital and valuable goal, that can improve your health and well-being, and save your life. Heart disease prevention is also a feasible and achievable goal, that can be accomplished by adopting healthy habits and behaviors, and using effective and proven methods and resources. Heart disease prevention is also a dynamic and evolving goal, that can be enhanced by following the latest trends and innovations, in science, technology, and medicine.

Heart disease is the leading cause of death and disability worldwide, affecting millions of people and their families. It is a complex and multifaceted condition that can be influenced by many factors, such as genetics, age, gender, ethnicity, and environment. However, it is also largely preventable and treatable, with the right knowledge, strategies, and actions. By reading this book, you have gained valuable information and insights that can help you take charge of your heart health and live a longer and happier life. However, this book is not meant to be a substitute for professional medical advice, diagnosis, or treatment. Always consult your doctor or health care provider before making any decisions or taking any actions regarding your heart health. Your doctor knows your medical history, condition, and needs, and can provide you with personalized and appropriate guidance and support. I hope that this book has inspired and motivated you to take action and improve your heart health. Remember, you are not alone in this journey. There are many resources and people that can help you along the way. Here are some of the additional resources and references that we recommend for further reading and learning:

1. American Heart Association

(https://www.heart.org/): A nonprofit organization that provides education, advocacy, and research on cardiovascular health and disease.

2. World Health Organization

(https://www.who.int/health-topics/cardiovascular-diseases#tab=tab_1): A specialized agency of the United Nations that provides global leadership and coordination on health issues, including heart disease.

3. Mayo Clinic

(https://www.mayoclinic.org/diseases-conditions/heart-disease/symptoms-causes/syc-20353118): A nonprofit academic medical center that offers comprehensive and reliable information and services on heart disease and other health topics.

4. Harvard Health Publishing

(https://www.health.harvard.edu/topics/heart-health): A division of Harvard Medical School that produces evidence-based and trustworthy content on heart health and wellness.

5. Heart Disease Prevention: From the Inside Out (https://www.amazon.com/Heart-Disease-Prevention-Inside-Out/dp/0984875511): A book by Dr. John M. Kennedy that explains the science and psychology of heart disease prevention and offers practical and holistic strategies for improving your heart health.

Special Bonus

Gain access to all my previous and future books

Please consider writing a review!